Newborn Life Support

5th Edition, May 2021

Reprinted October 2021

Reprinted June 2022

Reprinted January 2024

NLS

Newborn Life Support
5th Edition, May 2021

Reprinted October 2021
Reprinted June 2022
Reprinted January 2024

ISBN 978-1-903812-39-6

Published by © Resuscitation Council UK
1st Floor, 60-62 Margaret Street, London, W1W 8TF
Tel: 020 7388 4678 email: enquiries@resus.org.uk www.resus.org.uk

Printed by All About Print.
Tel: 020 7205 4022 email: hello@allaboutprint.co.uk www.allaboutprint.co.uk
Printed on responsibly sourced environmentally friendly paper made with elemental chlorine free fibre from legal and sustainably managed forests.

Photographs © Resuscitation Council UK

Photography by Ed Tyler and Ashley Prytherch
Colour plates reproduced with permission of the Northern Neonatal Network who retain copyright.

Design and artwork by Fruition London
www.fruitionlondon.com

The Resuscitation Council UK guidelines are adapted from the European Resuscitation Council guidelines and have been developed using a process accredited by The National Institute for Health and Care Excellence. The UK guidelines are consistent with the European guidelines but include minor modifications to reflect the needs of the National Health Service.

This Newborn Life Support (NLS) manual is written by Resuscitation Council UK NLS Subcommittee and forms part of the resources for Resuscitation Council UK NLS course, which is delivered in accredited course centres throughout the UK.

Acknowledgements

This text started life in the UK in 1980 as a small booklet written to help midwives, nurses and doctors faced, for the first time, with a responsibility for the care of babies at birth. Early editions were written by Dr Edmund Hey who, as a physiologist working with Professor Kenneth Cross in the 1960s, was involved in much of the original research into the physiology of neonatal asphyxia and temperature control. They were written to complement a regional theoretical and practical course in newborn resuscitation in the Northern Health Region of the United Kingdom. The booklet remained a locally written text, though with considerable national and a small international distribution, through a number of editions published by the Northern Neonatal Network. The fifth and final edition appeared in 1996. The working group is grateful to the Network for permission to reproduce their physiological diagrams. Dr Hey retired from his post as consultant neonatologist at the Princess Mary Maternity Hospital in Newcastle upon Tyne in 1994 and died in 2009.

When Resuscitation Council UK set up a working group to develop the Newborn Life Support course, Dr Sam Richmond, a long-time colleague and collaborator of Dr Hey, was appointed as chair. He was the editor of the first three versions of the NLS manual and closely involved in all aspects of the course and materials. Even after stepping down as chair, he remained involved as a member of the working group until shortly before his death in March 2013 and it is impossible to overestimate the loss of his giant intellect and encyclopaedic knowledge of the literature. He was also a chair of the NLS international Courses Committee of the European Resuscitation Council (ERC) and past co-chair of the neonatal task force of the International Liaison Committee on Resuscitation (ILCOR), evaluating evidence and writing guidelines from 2005 to 2010. He was made a Fellow of the ERC and an Honorary Member of Resuscitation Council UK in recognition of his contributions to resuscitation knowledge and training. The working group would all want to acknowledge his lasting contribution upon which this manual is built.

Professor Jonathan Wyllie was appointed NLS chair after Sam Richmond stepped down and steered the NLS course through resuscitation guideline revisions in 2010, 2015 and 2021. He edited the 4th edition of this manual and has a major role in international resuscitation science as previous vice-chair and emeritus member of the ILCOR NLS task force, Fellow of the ERC and President of Resuscitation Council UK. His wisdom and knowledge have shaped and enhanced the NLS manual and course materials.

We also would like to acknowledge the inspiration and constructive challenges afforded by regular meetings and conversations with Professors Jeffrey Perlman, John Kattwinkel, Myra Wyckoff and all the members of the neonatal section of the International Liaison Committee on Resuscitation (ILCOR) over the past 20 years. Any reader interested in exploring the evidence behind the various recommendations made in this and other texts on the topic of neonatal resuscitation are urged to access the evidence evaluations carried out in 2010, 2015 and 2021. There are hyperlinks in these documents to the relevant worksheets.

The URL is:

2020 https://doi.org/10.1016/j.resuscitation.2020.09.015

2015 http://www.resuscitationjournal.com/article/S0300-9572(15)00366-4/pdf

2010 http://circ.ahajournals.org/content/122/16_suppl_2/S516.full

We thank the Nuffield Hospital, Guildford, for the use of their facilities, the Royal Surrey NHS Foundation Trust, specifically the Resuscitation Department for their assistance with photography, Lifecast Body Simulation for the loan of manikins and all the Instructors who gave up their time to take part in the photography shoot.

We thank Ed Tyler and Ashley Prytherch for the photography taken and digitally prepared for the manual.

Finally, we would like to acknowledge the input, discussions and innovations in approach brought about by the interaction with the working group which developed the Advanced Resuscitation of the Newborn Infant (ARNI) course, especially the ARNI manual's editors, Drs Joe Fawke and Jonathan Cusack, and also Dr Fiona Wood for developments in teaching face mask ventilation.

Editors

Sean Ainsworth
Joe Fawke

Core editorial group

Sean Ainsworth
Adam Benson Clarke
Joe Fawke
Isabelle Hamilton-Bower
Sue Hampshire
John Madar
Vix Monnelly
Rob Tinnion
Jonathan Wyllie

Contributors

Joe Fawke
Sean Ainsworth
Adam Benson Clarke
T'ng Chang
Andy Coleman
Karen Cooper
Jonathan Cusack
John Goodinson
Isabelle Hamilton-Bower
Sue Hampshire
Katie Hunt
Hilary Lumsden
John Madar
Vix Monnelly
Eleri Pritchard
Alex Scrivens
Rachel Tennant
Rob Tinnion
Nicola Wenlock
Fiona Wood
Jonathan Wyllie

Contents

Contents

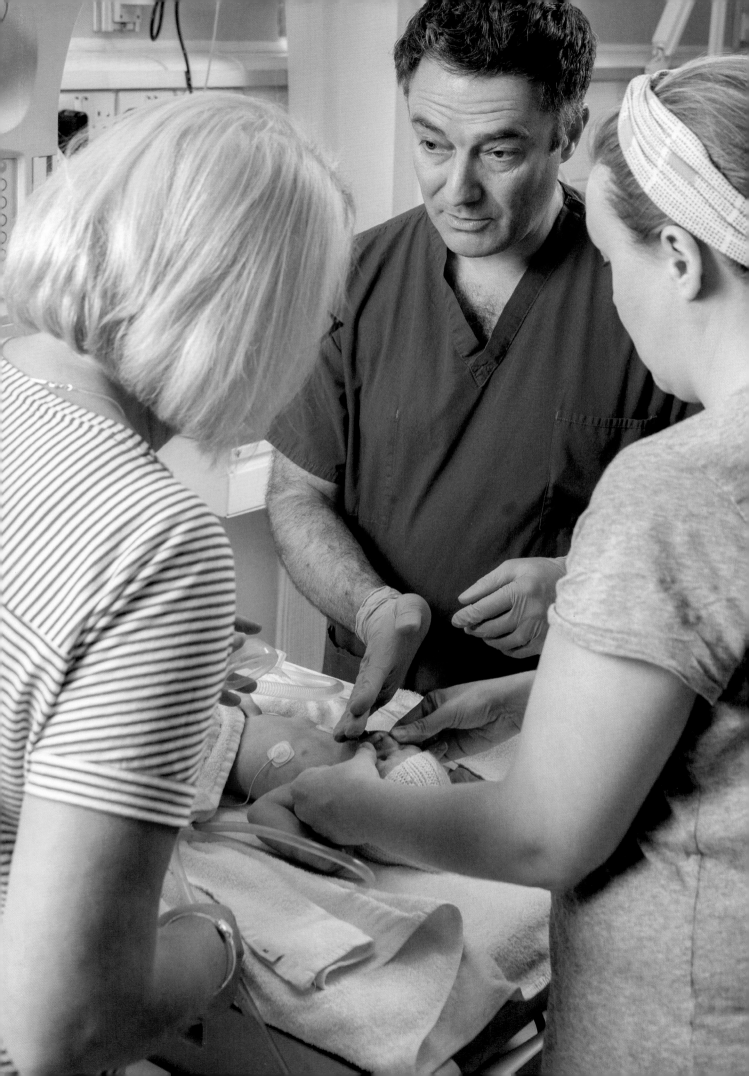

Introduction to the Newborn Life Support course

Aims of the NLS course

Once you have read the manual and completed the Newborn Life Support course, you should:

1. Understand the physiology and pathophysiology of transition at birth.

2. Be able to anticipate which babies may have problems, assess a baby at birth and recognise those who require additional help.

3. Be able to describe and follow a standardised approach to resuscitation or stabilisation at birth, emphasising the importance of thermal control and the priority of airway management and lung inflation and the limited role of chest compressions and drugs.

4. Have had practical experience in appropriate handling of the equipment used in newborn resuscitation.

5. Have learnt core skills in the management of the newborn airway, including strategies to help in situations where the initial attempt at lung inflation is unsuccessful.

6. Have been taught and practiced the following skills on manikins:

   a. Airway management, lung inflation and aeration

   b. Chest compressions

   c. Umbilical venous access.

7. Have been taught, practised and received constructive feedback about the immediate management of newborn emergencies in simulations with an appreciation of the importance of communication, human factors and teamwork.

8. Have demonstrated, in a test simulation using manikins, the core skills of thermal control, airway and breathing management of a newborn infant and subsequent, structured, management steps if initial attempts are unsuccessful.

9. Have developed a framework for succinct recording and effective communication of important details of the baby's condition at birth and the response to resuscitation.

10. Have practised the skills and developed an approach to newborn resuscitation during the first 10–20 min after birth as a basis to build upon with further mentored clinical training, which will permit achievement of clinical competence.

The Newborn Life Support (NLS) course has been developed, under the auspices of Resuscitation Council UK, to provide clear practical instruction in resuscitation of babies at birth. It is designed for all health workers who may be called upon to resuscitate a newborn baby, regardless of their discipline or status. The course is supported by the Royal College of Midwives, the British Association of Perinatal Medicine and the Royal College of Paediatrics and Child Health. It is kept up to date through an international collaborative cycle of evidence evaluation with the European Resuscitation Council and the International Liaison Committee on Resuscitation.

Why newborn babies are different and which need resuscitation

Introduction

Humans require immediate, life-saving assistance when breathing is interrupted, the circulation fails, or both. The immediate interventions that can be performed to aid recovery from this situation are generally termed 'resuscitation'. Birth is unique in that we are helping a baby start to breathe for the first time. Nonetheless, newborn babies are frequently reported as needing 'resuscitation' after birth. Sometimes this is the case but more often than not they just need assistance to transition to extrauterine life.

There are several differences between newborn babies compared with infants, children and adults. Not only are they smaller but they are also physiologically different and may need resuscitation for different reasons. A different approach to the resuscitation of a newborn baby is therefore necessary from that adopted with a collapsed child or adult.

Adults and children

In adults, collapse requiring resuscitation is usually due to a cardiac event, most commonly myocardial infarction, pulseless arrhythmia, or both. Breathing stops because oxygen is no longer being delivered to the respiratory centre in the brainstem. The resuscitator therefore has to reproduce the action of both the heart and the lungs in the hope of preserving flow of adequately oxygenated blood to the heart and brain. This is done using chest compressions and lung ventilation, usually referred to as cardiopulmonary resuscitation (CPR). The problem with the heart must be diagnosed and treated, usually requiring an ECG (or cardiac monitor), defibrillator and, occasionally, drugs. Throughout the time taken to do this, oxygen supply to the brain must be maintained using CPR to minimise subsequent neurological damage.

In children, collapse requiring resuscitation is usually respiratory in aetiology, which may lead to myocardial compromise and cardiac arrest. However, the underlying pathologies are many and varied.

Newborn babies

In newborn babies the problem is almost always one requiring primarily respiratory support. Being delivered through the birth canal is a hypoxic experience for the fetus because respiratory exchange via the placenta is interrupted for the 50–75 s duration of the average contraction. Whilst most babies tolerate this well, some do not and these few may require help to establish normal breathing.

The heart of the newborn baby can continue functioning for 20–30 min despite anoxia. The term newborn baby has evolved to undertake the strenuous passage through the birth canal and the brain of these babies can withstand lack of oxygen for much longer than an adult brain. During prolonged anoxia, however, the neural mechanisms driving attempts at normal breathing and the 'reserve' spinal reflex of anoxic gasping will cease to function if they are unsuccessful in drawing air into the lungs (Chapter 4).

To resuscitate a newborn baby, it is sufficient, in most cases, to aerate the lungs. Their lungs are initially fluid-filled, which makes the technique of initial lung aeration different. Whilst the fluid starts to be reabsorbed with the onset of labour, vaginally delivered babies at term still have about 100 mL of lung fluid to be absorbed. Those born by pre-labour caesarean section may have more fluid to clear.

In most cases of newborn 'resuscitation' the circulation is usually still functioning and 'aeration' or 'inflation' of the lungs will result in oxygenated blood returning to the heart from the lungs, leading to recovery. In rare instances the heart may need a brief period of chest compressions to achieve the same movement of oxygenated blood before the circulation is restored. The significant arrhythmias seen in adults do not occur, therefore the devices (e.g. defibrillators) needed to deal with these are unnecessary and even drugs are rarely needed.

Resuscitation or 'assisted transition'?

In adult medicine, the term 'resuscitation' is usually used to describe the urgent application of ventilation, chest compression, and often defibrillation, to an adult with no apparent signs of life.

Many discussions in the paediatric literature start with the unreferenced assertion that 'resuscitation' of the baby is necessary following 6 to 10% of all births. In the few studies that have examined this critically the need to apply both ventilation and chest compression to an apparently lifeless baby at birth is a rare event, occurring in about 1 in 2000 deliveries in countries with highly developed health care.[1] Approximately 85% of babies born at term will initiate spontaneous respirations within 10 to 30 s of birth; an additional 10% will respond during drying and stimulation, and approximately 3% will initiate respirations following positive pressure ventilation.[2,3] Crying can be a useful indicator as only babies who are breathing can cry. Breathing but non-crying babies may be slower to establish breathing with 9.5% not breathing until after 1 minute.[4]

In the context of newborn babies, the term 'resuscitation' is often used somewhat loosely. The babies that are clearly severely unwell at delivery and are, unarguably, in need of urgent attention to restore vital functions might legitimately be described as needing 'resuscitation'. However, this is not the usual experience of an attendant called to help a baby at delivery. In most cases, what's required is 'stabilisation' to assist the transition from placental to pulmonary respiration.[5] This is particularly true of the preterm infant where a hypoxic insult is not usually the primary issue.

Delayed cord clamping

Stable babies of any gestation who just need help with transitioning to extrauterine life benefit from delayed cord clamping. Practitioners need to plan how to achieve this (Chapter 6).

Keep babies warm

Babies are small and have a high surface-area-to-weight ratio. They are also born wet. These factors mean that babies can lose heat rapidly after birth, especially if receiving resuscitation. Specific measures are required to maintain the temperature in the normal range of 36.5°C to 37.5°C because hypothermia increases mortality and morbidity at all gestations. Although the focus is to keep the baby warm, hyperthermia may also be detrimental.

Airway and breathing

Prior to the development of the Newborn Life Support course, it was common for babies to be intubated; unnecessarily in many cases. One institution showed intubation rates fell from 7% to 1.5% following a change in policy, which had resulted in fewer deliveries being attended by a paediatrician.[6] Absence of a nationally agreed course and standard approach undoubtedly led to considerable, and occasionally injurious, variation in management; in the 1980s, 8–12% of newborn babies in one UK institution were intubated, whereas only 1.5–2% were at a comparable hospital in the same region.[7]

Information on the need for, rather than the receipt of, intubation comes from a study of over 95 000 births in Sweden.[8] A standard approach to resuscitation was taught that advocated mask inflation with progress to intubation only if mask inflation was unsuccessful. In babies weighing 2.5 kg or more, only about 10 babies per 1000 received mask inflation or intubation. Of these babies 8 per 1000 responded to mask inflation and only 2 per 1000 seemed to require intubation at birth. Similar data were obtained in a UK study of about 18 000 term deliveries over a four-year period which found that only 4 babies per 1000 were intubated.[9]

Equipment available for mask inflation 40 years ago was unsatisfactory, and lack of confidence was widespread, which probably explains the high intubation rates. There is little doubt that improved equipment[10] and training for mask ventilation[11] has helped reduce the need for intubation at birth.

Chest compressions and drugs

In adult resuscitation, the most effective intervention is usually defibrillation, with chest compressions being used to maintain a circulation to the brain and heart until such time as a defibrillator can be applied. In babies, the crucial intervention is to aerate and then ventilate the lungs.

Chest compression is needed only in a very few cases and then only to assist the heart in delivering oxygenated blood to the myocardium. The cartilaginous rib cage of the newborn and the larger size of the heart relative to the chest make chest compression much easier, as well as more efficient.

One American study over two years found only 39 (0.12%) of 30 839 infants received chest compressions and/or adrenaline (epinephrine) as part of cardiopulmonary resuscitation in the delivery room. Of these, 15 were term infants and 24 were premature.[12] In a 10 year retrospective review, the numbers of babies who needed full resuscitation (defined as requiring positive pressure ventilation via face mask and/or tracheal tube, cardiac compressions, and at least attempted central venous access for drugs) were very small; only 27 of approximately 60 000 babies met the criteria (i.e. less than 0.05%).[13]

Which deliveries should be attended by a practitioner trained in newborn resuscitation?

Many labour ward policies suggest the need for a practitioner trained in newborn resuscitation to attend a delivery is determined by the mode of delivery. This might demand attendance at all caesarean sections, all breech deliveries, all multiple deliveries, all instrumental deliveries, all preterm deliveries, all deliveries where monitoring (e.g. with cardiotocograph) suggests fetal compromise and all meconium staining. Such a policy would involve attending more than 30% of deliveries but would not eliminate the need for urgent calls to resuscitate babies found to be unexpectedly unresponsive at birth.[14] A more logical approach would be to relate the need to attend a delivery to the anticipated condition of the baby (Chapter 6).

Whatever guidelines are used to determine the presence of a practitioner trained in newborn resuscitation some babies will be born who unexpectedly require resuscitation. It is, therefore, particularly important that everyone who takes on the responsibility of delivering babies should be trained in resuscitation at birth and should undertake regular updates.

02: Summary learning

Babies are small and wet at birth and must be kept warm as hypothermia increases mortality.

A baby needing resuscitation at birth has a respiratory problem. Once air enters the lungs, the heart usually responds. Consequently, the most important skill to learn is that of effective airway management and successful lung aeration.

Most babies do not need resuscitation and breathe within 10–30 s of birth or after drying.

Of the 5% of babies who receive intervention, most respond after effective aeration of the lungs.

Most preterm infants merely require stabilisation to achieve transition not resuscitation.

My key take-home messages from this chapter are:

CPR - Cardiopulmonary Resuscitation
Adults - Cardiac event
Children - Respiratory
Vaginally born babies have 100ml of lung fluid
Pre labour CIS = more

"Resus" of the baby is necessary in 6-10% of births
Ventilation + Chest Compressions in 1:2000
85% of term babies will initiate spontaneous resps within 10-30 seconds
An additional 10% will respond during drying and simulation
3% following positive pressure ventilation

Delayed cord clamping helps the transition to extrauterine life

Intubation rates fell from 7% to 1.5% following the development of the NLS course

General care at birth

The learning outcomes will enable you to:

Describe the immediate management of newborn babies, including the majority who do not require any assistance with the transition to the extrauterine environment

Understand how to assess newborn babies to determine whether they need intervention or normal postnatal care

Introduction

Most mature babies will breathe or cry within 90 s of birth. Others need a little assistance, and it is expected that most babies will receive delayed umbilical cord clamping as standard care unless there is good reason not to do so. Very few newborn babies need resuscitation, even after an operative delivery. However, every newborn baby should be individually assessed at birth.

Initial actions at birth

The fetus respires via the placenta. After birth, this function is taken over by the lungs. Following normal birth, a transition from one method of respiration to the other occurs. This can take a few minutes to complete, though in most instances it happens very quickly. While this is happening, redistribution of blood between the placenta and the baby is also occurring. In a healthy baby there is no need to interrupt this process by clamping the cord. It is important to assess the baby at delivery to determine how to manage the clamping of the cord; can it be delayed or do you need to consider another approach? Delayed cord clamping is covered in detail in Chapter 6.

Assessment should be accompanied by gentle stimulation, such as drying or rubbing with a towel. Methods of tactile stimulation vary widely and the optimal method remains unknown.[15,16] The benefits seem to be greater in preterm babies than in term babies.[17] If your assessment determines the baby is healthy, delay clamping the cord for at least 60 s (ideally until after breathing is established) whilst keeping the baby warm.[18] To prevent heat loss, the baby can be wrapped, and if placed skin-to-skin should also be covered. It is worth remembering that blood gained from the placenta is at maternal body temperature and may help keep the baby warm.[19]

It is not necessary to spend time trying to remove small amounts of liquor from the mouth and nose because the average 3.5 kg baby will clear about 100 mL of fluid from the lungs and trachea unaided in a matter of minutes.[20,21] They do not need to be subjected to vigorous suction but should be dried and wrapped in dry towels to minimise heat loss.

Warmth: maintaining normothermia

Keeping the baby warm is essential because getting cold increases the risk of death or serious morbidity. Because of their small size and relatively large surface area, babies can get cold very quickly. The human fetus has a higher temperature (approximately 0.5°C) than its mother[22] and can become very cold very quickly after birth without active management. One baby, born by an unattended delivery at home, was reported to have a core temperature of 18°C when admitted to hospital 40 min after delivery.[23] Even in a delivery room, if left naked and wet, the baby's temperature can fall to 33°C within 5 min.[24] Ideally the baby should be born into an environment that is warm enough to allow it to maintain a body temperature within the normal range without effort.

Newborn babies subjected to cold stress have a lower oxygen tension[25] and a worse metabolic acidosis.[26] Animal model evidence suggests that hypoxia, acidosis and hypothermia all inhibit surfactant production.[27]

The admission temperature of newly born babies is a strong predictor of mortality and morbidity at all gestations, especially in very small and preterm babies [28-30] and should be recorded as a predictor of outcome as well as a quality indicator.[31] Hypothermia is associated with increased mortality and morbidity especially in small and preterm babies.[29] For every 1°C below 36.5°C the baseline risk of mortality increases by up to 28% in very low birth weight babies.[32]

During resuscitation and immediately afterwards, the temperature of all newborn babies should be maintained between 36.5°C and 37.5°C. In some babies, therapeutic hypothermia may be started once the appropriate assessments for this have been completed (usually in a neonatal unit environment).[33]

Methods of heat loss

Heat loss occurs by four different routes: evaporation, convection, conduction and radiation. When the skin is wet with amniotic fluid, moisture quickly evaporates from the skin's surface taking a large amount of heat with it as latent heat of evaporation. Draughts of air moving past the baby encourage this and also cause loss of heat by convection. Placing the baby on a cold surface such as cool mattresses or towels will risk heat loss by conduction. Finally, the baby may lose heat by radiation from uncovered skin surfaces direct to cooler surfaces. In the newborn baby most heat is lost by evaporation and convection.

Preventing heat loss

There are several simple and effective ways by which heat loss can be kept to a minimum:

- Dry the baby and wrap in a pre-warmed towel to prevent evaporative heat loss.[34] Use a hat to cover the head.
- Keep the delivery area draught free by keeping doors and windows shut wherever possible, to reduce heat loss by convection.
- Maintain the environmental temperature within the range 23–25°C.[35,36]
- Place the baby skin-to-skin and cover.[37]
- If the baby needs attention use a radiant heater to reduce heat loss by radiation and conduction.

Preterm babies are particularly vulnerable to heat loss which can be reduced by using a plastic bag (Figure 3.1). It is likely that a combination of methods will be required to maintain the temperature in babies who are either premature or who require help (Chapter 9).

Figure 3.1   Using warm dry towels, a plastic bag and a hat to reduce heat loss in a preterm baby. A heat source will also be required.

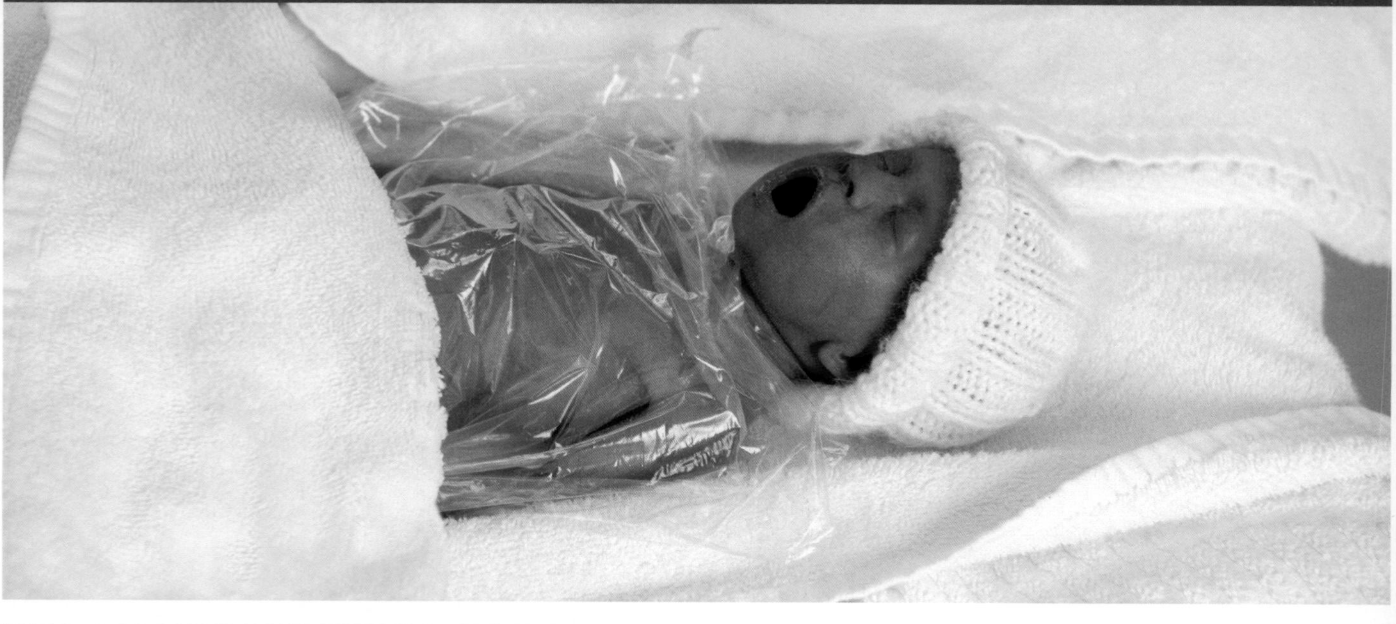

Assessment of the newborn

Whilst the umbilical cord is intact an initial assessment of the baby should occur. During this time keep the baby warm and assess:

| colour |
| tone |
| breathing |
| heart rate |

The items are listed in this order because this is the order in which this information becomes available. Colour can be assessed as soon as you see the baby, tone can be appreciated when you see and touch the baby, breathing can be noted almost as quickly, but detection of heart rate requires a little more time, and usually the use of a stethoscope. Reassess heart rate and breathing regularly during any subsequent resuscitation, as these are the first to change and can be used to guide your actions.

Colour

Look at the colour of the trunk, lips and tongue. Most babies appear blue at first and can remain so for several minutes after birth; this alone does not mean the baby requires assistance. Other elements of the assessment are needed to fully guide any interventions.

Tone

Note whether the baby is well flexed with good tone, or floppy.

Breathing

Look at the rate and pattern of breathing. Most babies will breathe or cry within 30 s of birth and establish regular respirations by 60 s.[4] Without intervention such as drying, stimulation and beginning lung inflation, up to 20% of healthy babies may take 60–180 s to establish regular breathing.[38] Gasping respirations are usually a sign that the baby will need help.

Heart rate

For most delivery situations, checking the heart rate with a stethoscope will provide an inexpensive, simple and readily available accurate estimate of heart rate. In an apnoeic baby the slow pulsation of the ventricles may be seen lifting the chest wall. The cord may pulsate; however this is not reliable as pulsations are not always present, even in a healthy baby, and the rate of cord pulsation does not always reflect the actual heart rate. If you feel pulsations of over 100 min[-1] in the cord it suggests all is well, but the reverse is not true for slower or an absent cord pulse rate.[39]

Continuous monitoring provides a more dynamic indication of heart rate change during resuscitation and is preferable to intermittent counting; both pulse oximetry and ECG are available and can be very useful in longer resuscitations.

Interpretation

A baby who is initially blue but breathing regularly, with a fast heart rate, and who has good tone, needs no further intervention (other than to maintain its temperature) and may be given to the mother. A further assessment should be made of the colour to check this is continuing to improve but if the baby is breathing regularly this need not involve anything more than a quick visual check.

A baby who is not breathing adequately with a slow heart rate, or who is blue-white or floppy, should be dried and covered and where possible use a radiant heat source. Further actions may then be taken. This may require the umbilical cord to be clamped and cut, interrupting delayed cord clamping, if not already done by the birth attendant.

> Call for help if you or the situation (as assessed above) require it

Care of the baby who requires no further help

Parents

At delivery, do not take the baby away from the mother unless this is clearly necessary. Both parents may want to hold their baby and, if the baby appears well, they should be encouraged to do so once their baby has been dried and wrapped. The baby should be kept warm and this is also a very good time to initiate breastfeeding. The risk of mature babies becoming cold while they remain in the warmth of their mother's arms is very low, even if unclothed (skin-to-skin), as long as the mother and baby are protected from draughts by a blanket, the baby has been dried, and the environment is warm (Figure 3.2).[34,37]

Early feeding

All babies experience a physiological fall in blood glucose in the first few hours after birth. The lowest point of this fall can reach levels of 1–2 mmol L[-1]. This level in adults would cause unconsciousness or even fitting but does not do so in appropriately grown, well, term newborn babies because alternative fuels for the brain are usually easily available in the form of lactate and ketones. Lactate can be relatively high at birth and falls in the first few hours, thus providing alternative brain fuel while blood glucose production from glycogen is initiated.[40] Within a few hours of birth, most babies start to produce ketones which can also be used as brain fuel and which will be available for the first 72 hours or so while breastfeeding becomes established.[40]

Preterm babies and babies who are small for gestational age are less able to produce this protective ketogenic response.[41] Infants of insulin-dependent diabetic mothers may have a higher requirement for glucose.[42] Some maternal medications may also impair a baby's ability to maintain their blood sugar.[43] Babies who get cold, and thus have to use energy to try to maintain their body temperature, will use up their fuel reserves more rapidly. There is no need to wash the baby at birth. Doing so makes the baby very cold unnecessarily.[34]

Preventing sudden unexpected postnatal collapse

Respect the family's need for peace and privacy but ensure that the baby's airway is not compromised especially as many are placed prone on their mother's chest during skin-to-skin care, a position not recommended at any other time due to increased risks of airway obstruction.[44]

Sudden unexpected postnatal collapse (SUPC) is a rare event in term or near-term babies who are otherwise well at birth and who are assigned to routine postnatal care. These babies collapse unexpectedly and require resuscitation.[45] Although rare, there is a consistent and concerning observation that SUPC occurs in the context of skin-to-skin care and breastfeeding, particularly when prone.[46] Worry about SUPC should not prevent skin-to-skin care or early breastfeeding but enhanced vigilance during these activities may be important in preventing SUPC.[46]

Examination

The baby should be briefly examined shortly after birth and in the presence of the parents. This examination should check for any signs of cardio-respiratory distress, major congenital anomalies, birthmarks or birth injuries. The baby must be kept warm during this process and all findings should be recorded in the baby notes. A more detailed examination will take place later.

Figure 3.2 Baby skin-to-skin, covered, in a supported position, but without head covering. Attention should also be paid to the temperature in the room.

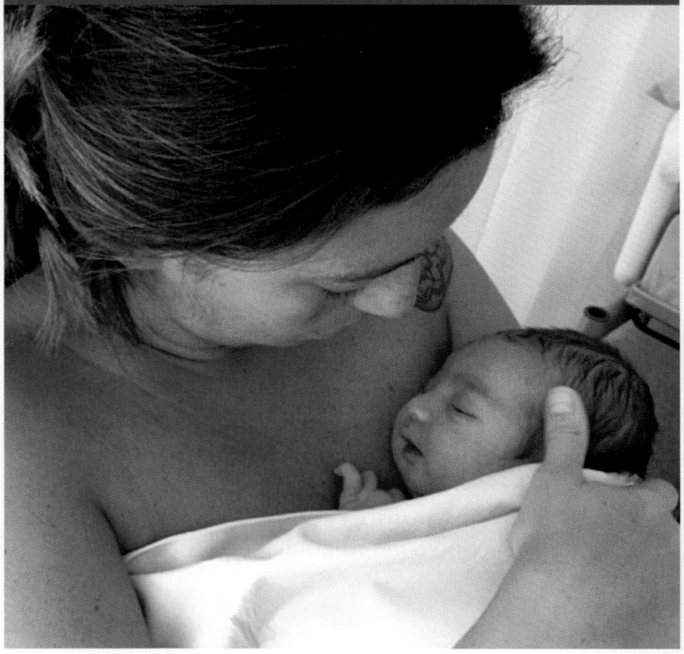

03: Summary learning

An initial assessment of the baby's condition can be made quickly after birth.

Allow time for placental transfusion, by delaying umbilical cord clamping for at least 60 s unless immediate resuscitation is required.

The importance of drying and covering the baby to prevent heat loss cannot be over emphasised.

Do not take the baby away from the parents unless it is clearly necessary.

My key take-home messages from this chapter are:

- Following birth a transition between one method of respiration and another occurs. While this happens, redistribution of blood between the placenta and baby also occurs
- Baby temp is about 0.5°C warmer than its mother
- Surfactant production is inhibited by hypoxia, acidosis + hypothermia
- For every 1°C below 36.5°C the base line risk of mortality increases by up to 28% in very low BW babies
- During resus and immediately afterwards the temp of a newborn should be maintained between 36.5° + 37.5°
- HEAT LOSS OCCURS BY –
  * Evaporation – wet skin
  * Convection – draughts
  * Conduction – placing baby on cold surface
  * Radiation – uncovered skin directly on cooler surfaces
- Reduce heat loss in preterm babies by using a plastic bag

Introduction

Transition from the intrauterine to extrauterine environment is a complex physiological event. In most cases, the process leads to the successful transition from fetal dependence on placental respiration to a baby breathing air. Understanding the process of normal transition and how this might go wrong, as well as what happens during resuscitation, provides us with a logical approach to stabilisation and resuscitation. It helps explain the importance of what we do, and the order in which we do it.

Terms used

Many of the terms used to describe the events during the transition to air breathing carry medico-legal as well as pathophysiological implications. Unfortunately, the terms have been used quite interchangeably, and somewhat loosely, in the past.

The following is a list of terms that may be found in texts and papers on the subject:

Acidaemia	Increased concentration of hydrogen ions in blood
Acidosis	Although the term is frequently used interchangeably with acidaemia, acidosis is the process leading to increased concentration of hydrogen ions in any tissue. • A respiratory acidosis arises when there is an accumulation of carbon dioxide (which is converted into carbonic acid). • A metabolic acidosis arises when there is an accumulation of acids that arise from the body's metabolism (such as lactic acid, which is produced as a by-product of anaerobic metabolism, or any one of a number of organic acids that accumulate in inherited metabolic conditions). A mixed acidosis has both respiratory and other components.
Anoxia	Complete lack of oxygen in any tissue
Asphyxia	A condition in which an extreme decrease in the concentration of oxygen in the body leads to loss of consciousness or death. There may or may not be an accompanying increase in carbon dioxide. In most cases asphyxia arises due to the interruption of gas exchange however restriction of cerebral blood flow may also lead to cerebral hypoperfusion and hypoxia. The term is best avoided, having been replaced in the mid-twentieth century by more specific terms such as anoxia, hypoxia, hypoxaemia, hypercapnia.
Hypercapnia (also hypercarbia)	Abnormally high levels of carbon dioxide in the blood.
Hypoxaemia	Decreased oxygen content of blood.
Hypoxia	Decreased level of oxygen in any tissue.

Historical approaches to resuscitation

Until the late 1950s, resuscitation at birth had never been subjected to systematic study. Numerous techniques such as intragastric oxygen,[48-50] the dropping of respiratory stimulant drugs on the tongue,[51-53] Eve's rocking method,[54-56] hyperbaric oxygen[57,58] and rapid hypothermia[59,60] were widely advocated and employed with apparent success. All these techniques are now discredited and several have been shown to be harmful. Although therapeutically-induced hypothermia in the post-resuscitation period has been shown to be useful in reducing long-term neurological damage after significant damaging hypoxia in term babies,[61] it is of no help during resuscitation and harmful in all other situations. Furthermore, more than 90% of the babies subjected to these historical treatments survived, which is a vivid testimony to the fact that most newborn babies have remarkable powers of recovery.

Thanks to the work undertaken by Geoffrey Dawes in Oxford,[62] Kenneth Cross in London,[63] and several other neonatal physiologists[64], we now have a much better understanding of the sequence of events which occur when mammals are subjected to acute hypoxia during birth. These studies also inform a logical and effective response. Much of what we know about the subject was learnt between 1957 and 1967 – a decade that witnessed a complete transformation in the way newborn babies were resuscitated. That knowledge is currently being supplemented using information obtained from both animal and human studies during birth using newer investigative techniques to enhance our understanding of both normal and abnormal transition at birth.[65-69]

Coincident with advances in the knowledge about the physiology came changes in resuscitation techniques; adult mouth-to-mouth resuscitation was described in 1958,[70] and the complementary technique of closed-chest cardiac compression two years later.[71] Within a year there were reports of the latter technique being successfully used on a baby.[72] Tracheal intubation came to be widely adopted in the 1960s[73,74] even though this approach had been strongly recommended as early as 1928.[75]

Physiology of normal transition

Birth represents a significant physiological challenge for a fetus: changing from a liquid-filled intrauterine environment to independent life in air.[76,77] Surprisingly, most babies undergo this change without apparent difficulty but some babies, particularly those born prematurely, require assistance most commonly in the form of respiratory support.[76]

A. Fetal respiration and circulation

During fetal life, the lungs are liquid-filled and therefore play no part in gas exchange, which occurs across the placenta.[78,79] Pulmonary arterial resistance is high and so right-to-left shunting of blood occurs through the ductus arteriosus and the foramen ovale. In contrast the placental bed, which is fed through the systemic circulation, has a relatively low vascular resistance.

The fetal systemic circulation is fed from both the left and right ventricles. The average combined ventricular output in the near-term fetus is 465 mL kg min^{-1}; about 55% of this is from the right ventricle, and 45% from the left. About 75% of right ventricular output flows through the ductus arteriosus to supply the abdomen, lower body and the placenta and about 75% of left ventricular output perfuses the upper body (head, neck, and arms). The remaining 25% mixes with the output from the other ventricle.[80] The blood flow to the placenta increases with increasing fetal maturity (17% of the combined ventricular output at 10 weeks increasing to 33% at 20 weeks of gestation[81]) until near-term, where it decreases to around 22–26%.[82]

B. Antenatal preparation for birth

i. Fetal lung fluid

Fetal lung fluid is produced by the epithelial lining of the developing lung and because of the resistance imparted by laryngeal abduction it plays a critical role in fetal lung growth and development by maintaining the lungs in a distended state. Production of fetal lung fluid increases with increasing gestational age, and as the fetus approaches term it accumulates to a total volume of 20–30 mL kg^{-1} (equivalent to the functional residual capacity). If insufficient amniotic fluid and consequently fetal lung fluid is present, then lung development can be adversely affected causing pulmonary hypoplasia.

The process of labour stimulates production of adrenaline by the fetus[83] and thyrotropin releasing hormone by the mother.[84] This encourages the alveolar cells responsible for secreting lung fluid in the fetus to cease production and to begin to absorb fluid from the alveolar spaces, preparing the lungs for air breathing. How this is achieved is variable and different mechanisms almost certainly co-exist.

The clearance of fetal lung fluid by epithelial sodium channels appears important in some animals[85] but the effect in humans is less convincing. It is also less likely to occur in preterm babies as the mechanism for reabsorption matures only late in gestation.[86]

ii. Fetal breathing and its relationship to breathing after birth

Movements of the fetal chest (erroneously called fetal breathing) are essential for normal lung growth and can be detected as early as 10 weeks' gestation. With increasing maturity, such movements occur more often; they are present for 10–20% of the time at 24 to 28 weeks and increase to 30–40% after 30 weeks. Each period of fetal lung movements is also sustained for longer. Despite this the volume of lung fluid moved during each 'breath' is small and insufficient to be cleared from the trachea; these fetal lung movements, therefore, play little or no part in the preparation for birth.

The initiation of breathing after birth is complex and poorly understood. Prior to birth, the carotid body, the main peripheral arterial chemoreceptor responsible for stimulating the body's response to hypoxia, hypercapnia and acidosis, is relatively insensitive.[87,88] In addition, breathing of the quality and quantity seen after birth is inhibited by prostaglandin E_2 produced by the placenta.[89]

C. Intrapartum events in relation to placental and fetal blood flow and impact on gas exchange

Before the onset of labour, the fetus exists in a hypoxaemic state; the average partial pressure in umbilical venous blood is 7.3 kPa; that in the umbilical artery (and thus representative of oxygen supply to the tissues) is 4.53 kPa whereas partial pressure of the mother's arterial oxygen is typically 13.3 kPa.[90]

During labour, recurrent uterine contractions may transiently interfere with uterine arterial blood flow and placental gas exchange.[91] In uncomplicated labour this is generally of little or no consequence for the fetus.[92] Labour may be less well tolerated by fetuses with other issues e.g. sepsis or growth restriction.

However, if the hypoxia continues, or the placental blood flow is reduced[89] or if the cord is obstructed[93,94] the fetus then begins to follow the sequence of events described later in this chapter.

D. Establishing breathing at birth

At birth, the lungs must take over the role of the gas exchange organ. To achieve this, the alveoli must be aerated and blood flow through the lungs must increase significantly.[77,95]

In the healthy newborn, both skin stimulation and skin cooling (in the absence of core temperature changes) stimulate respiration.[94,96] Whilst a difference in core and surface temperature may stimulate the initiation of breathing, it is essential that a baby's core temperature is maintained in the normal range (Chapter 5). If the airway is open, those first few breaths aerate the lungs[21] and continuous breathing is established. Clearance of fetal lung fluid and the formation of a large well-perfused gas exchange surface is essential.

Although there is a suggestion that small amounts of fetal lung fluid might be absorbed prior to delivery, slightly more is lost from the upper airways during cephalic vaginal delivery. It was originally thought that the 'vaginal squeeze' associated with normal delivery was a major contributing factor but it is now realised that the human thorax does not represent a large volume within the birth canal.[97] Instead, it seems more likely that it is postural changes imposed on the fetus during uterine contractions that contribute to loss of some lung liquid via upper airways.[77]

Furthermore, it is now understood that the primary mechanism for airway liquid clearance after birth, and thus responsible for clearance of most fetal lung fluid, lies with the hydrostatic pressures generated by inspiration.[66,98] Spontaneous inspiratory movements by the newborn baby generate a transepithelial pressure gradient between the interstitial tissue and airway lumen, and as a result the lung fluid is drawn from the proximal airways into distal ones where it is cleared across the distal airway wall into the surrounding interstitial tissue space.[99] In term babies, these spontaneous breaths can generate intrathoracic pressures of between -20 and -80 cm water.[100]

Phase-contrast x-ray imaging of the pattern of air entry into the lungs of spontaneously breathing term newborn rabbits demonstrate that lung aeration mostly (~95%) occurs during inspiration, with no liquid clearance occurring between breaths.[66,101] The movement of liquid across the epithelium is extremely rapid, resulting in almost complete airway liquid clearance (> 15 mL kg⁻¹ of liquid) during the breaths in the first 15–30 s.

As the fluid enters the interstitial tissue it causes the hydrostatic pressure in that tissue to rise to approximately 6 cm water,[102] driving some fluid back into the airway, especially during expiration. This liquid is quickly re-cleared during subsequent inspirations, resulting in a continuous cycle of airway liquid clearance and partial re-entry during the breathing cycle and there is a progressive aeration of airway from proximal to distal.[64]

Because the viscosity of liquid is considerably higher than air, the resistance is ~100 times greater when the lung is liquid-filled versus when it is air-filled. As the airways progressively open, resistance decreases and pulmonary compliance increases rapidly.[103] Clearance of this lung fluid from interstitial tissue via lymphatics and blood vessels takes considerably longer (4–6 hours). During this time the pressure in the interstitial tissue, which has risen to approximately 6 cm water during the first few breaths, gradually decreases.[102]

In healthy newborn babies, lung ultrasound shows that lung aeration and partial airway liquid clearance is achieved within the first 20 minutes and complete airway liquid clearance is typically achieved within 4 hours.[67] The first few breaths do not usually result in gas exchange and it takes a median of 7 breaths before exhaled carbon dioxide can be detected in spontaneously breathing babies. The exhaled carbon dioxide peaks in the first 2–3 minutes after birth (coinciding with increased tidal volumes and respiratory rates) before settling down to a post-transitional plateau.[104] Tidal volumes generated by the baby (i.e. the volume of air within each breath) during these first few minutes can reach a median volume of 19 mL kg^{-1} before settling to a median of 5.8 mL kg^{-1}.[104]

E. Pulmonary blood flow, cardiac output and cord clamping

Aeration of the lungs triggers a decrease in pulmonary vascular resistance and an increase in pulmonary blood flow. Whilst lung expansion is the primary driver for the increase in pulmonary blood flow the exact mechanisms governing this event remain unclear.[105] What is clear is that the timing of the clamping of the umbilical cord is important.

In the fetus, the placenta provides 30–50% of the venous return to the heart; immediate clamping of the cord instantly reduces the venous return by this amount whilst at the same time bringing about a rise in systemic vascular resistance by removing the low resistance placental circulation from the systemic portion of the circulation.[106] Within 4 cardiac cycles this causes both a 30% increase in systemic blood pressure and a 30–50% decrease in cardiac output. The cardiac output remains low until lung aeration and ventilation occurs and the pulmonary blood flow begins to increase. In turn, this then causes the flow to the left atrium to increase.[106,107]

Observational studies of heart rate at birth in normal healthy babies following immediate cord clamping show a reduction in heart rates after birth increasing within a few minutes,[108] a finding first published more than 60 years ago by Brady and James[109] and by Lind and colleagues[110-112] although the importance of the effect of immediate cord clamping was largely ignored at that time by the wider clinical community. In 1981, one of Lind's colleagues[113] recalled how at the 1959 Scandinavian Congress of Physiologists a cineradiography of the first breath was shown; and that

"if the umbilical cord is tied prior to the first breath, the result is a decrease in the size of the heart during the first three or four cardiac cycles. Then the heart again increases in size, almost to that of the fetal heart".

This decrease in venous return seen with immediate clamping of the umbilical cord can be avoided by increasing the pulmonary blood flow; if the baby breathes and the lungs expand before the umbilical cord is clamped, venous return will be maintained, in part, by umbilical venous return. At the same time the shunting through the ductus arteriosus changes from the fetal right-to-left pattern to a left-to-right pattern that contributes a further 30–50% to pulmonary blood flow during the first 10 minutes after birth.[114] Induced bradycardia is thereby avoided.

With an intact umbilical cord, the transition from umbilical venous return to pulmonary venous return is smoother and fluctuations in systemic arterial blood pressure and pulmonary blood flow are reduced.[106] When cord clamping is delayed until after babies breathe the initial bradycardia is not seen.[115] Term babies who breathe spontaneously and do not have their cord clamped for 5 minutes, gain on average 116 grams in weight (equivalent to 110 mL of blood) during this time.[116]

Table 4.1 A summary of the many causes of peripartum diseases and conditions that can lead to fetal or infant cerebral anoxia

Maternal conditions	Placental or umbilical cord problems	Fetal and postnatal problems
Hypertension	Placental abruption[118]	Congenital airway abnormalities
Pre-eclampsia	Feto-maternal haemorrhage	Central hypoventilation
Hypotensive shock	Umbilical cord compression	Severe cardiopulmonary disease
Uterine rupture[117]	– Cord prolapse[119]	Hypovolaemia
Sepsis	– Nuchal cord[120]	Hydrops fetalis
Severe anaemia	– True knot	Sepsis
	Velamentous cord insertion[121]	Maternal medications

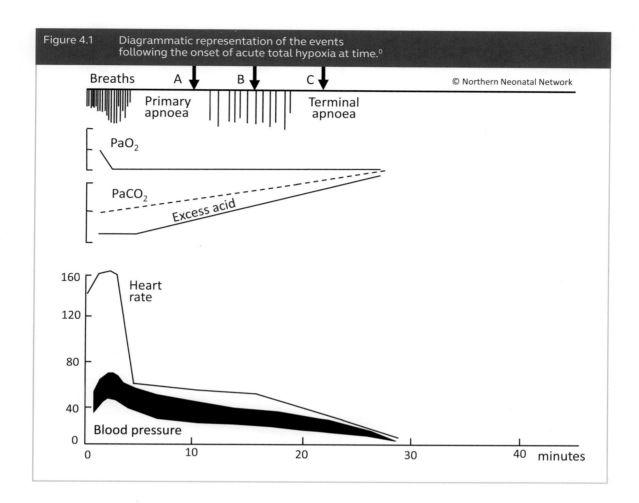

Figure 4.1 Diagrammatic representation of the events following the onset of acute total hypoxia at time.[0]

© Northern Neonatal Network

The pathophysiology of abnormal transition/maladaptation

A. Causes of abnormal transition

Interruption of the placental blood flow is the most frequent final pathway leading to perinatal hypoxia. There are many factors that can contribute to this (Table 4.1).

Interruption of placental blood flow provokes several adaptive mechanisms in the fetus. The understanding of these comes from animal studies of acute intrapartum hypoxia. Whilst there are differences between human and other mammalian anatomy, the physiological responses to both interupted placental blood flow and resuscitation measures are consistent across all species studied so far.

B. Fetal response to acute hypoxia and other insults

Figures 4.2 to 4.3 show data derived from animal experiments outlining the response of an intrauterine mammalian fetus subjected to acute total hypoxia.[62] These data were obtained by opening the pregnant uterus of a mammal in such a way as to avoid uterine contraction, then preventing the fetus from being able to aerate its lungs by placing its head in a bag of sodium chloride, and finally obstructing the fetoplacental circulation.

At the onset of acute hypoxia and hypercapnia the conscious fetus' breathing movements, driven by the respiratory centre, become deeper and more rapid. During this time the PaO_2 falls rapidly and soon the fetus loses consciousness. Within a few minutes, regular breathing movements cease as the higher centres (especially the respiratory centre) responsible for controlling them are unable to continue to function due to lack of oxygen and the fetus enters a period known as primary apnoea. Up to this point the heart rate has been maintained but soon falls to about half its normal rate, though the blood pressure is almost unchanged.

The initial fall in heart rate is probably a vagally-induced event, but this slow rate continues because a lack of oxygen means the heart uses less fuel efficient anaerobic metabolism to function. This is possible in the newborn because, at term, the heart and liver have stores of glycogen that can be utilised during anaerobic metabolism. Blood pressure is maintained despite a lower heart rate because vasoconstriction restricts flow to all but the most vital areas.

At the same time, the slower heart rate allows more time for the ventricles to refill during diastole and the stroke volume (i.e. the volume of blood ejected during a single contraction) increases slightly. Thus overall, cardiac output drops due to the slower heart rate but the fall is not as great as would be predicted from the fall in rate alone. By these methods, the circulation is maintained to the organs of the body that are most important for immediate survival but at a cost of further deterioration of the biochemical milieu due to the release of lactic acid as a by-product of anaerobic metabolism.

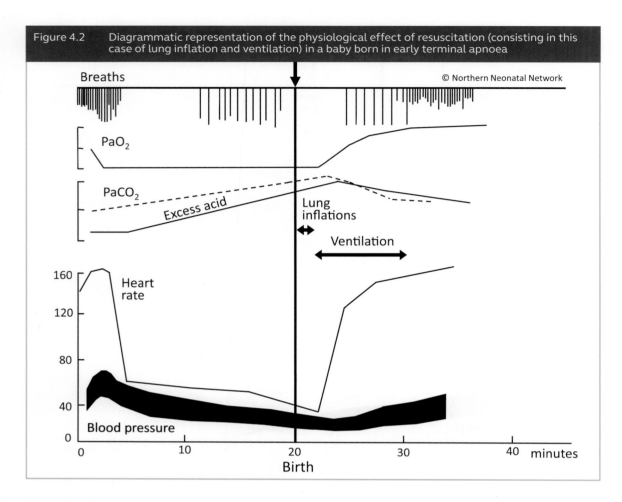

Figure 4.2 Diagrammatic representation of the physiological effect of resuscitation (consisting in this case of lung inflation and ventilation) in a baby born in early terminal apnoea

© Northern Neonatal Network

If the hypoxia continues, and the fetus is not delivered, then after a variable period of time, primitive spinal centres (released from suppression by the higher breathing centres) produce shuddering whole body gasps at a rate of about 12 min^{-1}.[62] A variable time may elapse before this unconscious, reflex, gasping activity begins. Anaesthetics and drugs, especially opiates, given to the mother can increase the duration of this primary apnoeic period but the length of the following period of gasping is then reduced.[122]

During this period of gasping some cardiopulmonary circulation is maintained but if these gasps fail to aerate the lungs they fade away as increasing acidosis together with the hypoxia interferes with synaptic communication between nerve cells[53] and the fetus enters terminal apnoea. Soon, the rapidly deteriorating biochemical milieu, with profound metabolic and respiratory acidosis as well as hypoxia causes the heart muscle to cease to function effectively and, without further intervention, the baby dies. The whole process probably takes almost thirty minutes in the newborn human baby.[123]

C. Response to resuscitation

i. Self-resuscitating babies (i.e. primary apnoea and during agonal gasps)

A baby who is not breathing within 1–2 minutes of birth could have reached one of the three points indicated by arrows in Figure 4.1. It is not usually possible to confidently assess at this stage whether the baby is born at the point of the first, second or third arrow.

A baby born at the point indicated by the first arrow will be perfectly able to 'resuscitate' itself provided the airway is clear. After a pause this baby will take the first of a series of gasps. If the airway is open and these gasps are successful in aerating the lungs then, because the circulation is still functioning, blood oxygenated by the aerated lungs will be transported to the coronary arteries and the heart rate will increase.

The improving circulation will then, in turn, transport oxygenated blood to the brain and the respiratory centre. Once the respiratory centre is functioning again, normal regular breathing will start and gasping will cease. A similar sequence of events will follow in a baby born at the second arrow, though recovery may be somewhat slower. The baby who has reached the point indicated by the third arrow will certainly die without intervention and may even die despite it.

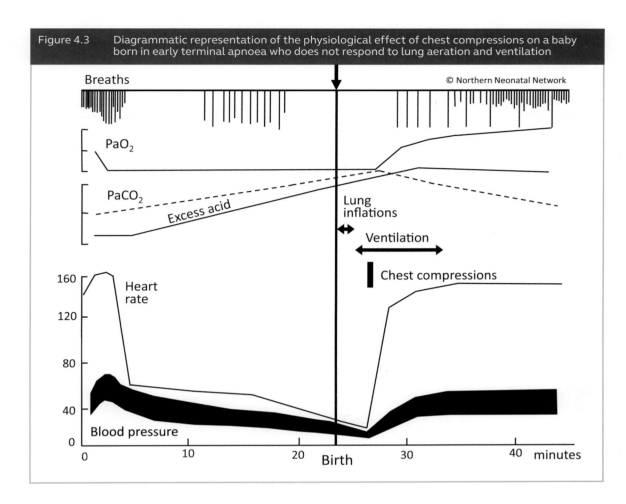

Figure 4.3 Diagrammatic representation of the physiological effect of chest compressions on a baby born in early terminal apnoea who does not respond to lung aeration and ventilation

ii. Resuscitation of babies in terminal apnoea

Effective lung aeration may be enough to produce a rapid recovery, provided the circulation is functioning sufficiently to bring some oxygenated blood back to the heart (Figure 4.2). Unfortunately, it is not possible to tell at the time whether a baby who is not breathing at birth is in primary apnoea and about to gasp or whether it has already taken its last gasp before being born. It is reassuring to know, however, that almost all babies for whom help is called at birth will respond very rapidly once their lungs are aerated.

Figure 4.2 shows such a response to resuscitation from a baby in early terminal apnoea. A similar response would be expected had the baby been born in primary apnoea (arrow 1; Figure 4.1) but in that case one would expect few, if any gasps, following lung aeration. The baby who was resuscitated from primary apnoea would have been more likely to breathe normally.

In a few babies, the situation may have progressed to a stage where the heart rate shows no response. In this case the heart is no longer able to deliver oxygenated blood from the lungs to the coronary arteries despite adequate lung aeration and subsequent ventilation. In this situation, recovery may still occur if a brief period of chest compressions can successfully deliver a small quantity of oxygenated blood to the heart, provided the heart is still able to respond as is illustrated opposite (Figure 4.3). This may need to be followed by a period of ventilation breaths until normal breathing is established.

As previously stated, it is impossible to tell at the time whether an apnoeic baby at birth is in primary apnoea and about to gasp or whether they have already taken their last gasp before being born and is now in terminal apnoea. The NLS approach has been developed to cope equally well with either situation. Such an approach is outlined in the next chapter.

04: Summary learning

Most babies make the transition to extrauterine life independently and without difficulty by embarking on a sequence of respiratory and cardiovascular changes during the first few minutes after birth.

Immediate clamping of the cord may produce initial bradycardia, which then resolves. In babies who do not require resuscitation, unless there are clear reasons not to do so, the cord should not be clamped for at least 60 s and ideally not until after respirations are established.

There are three reasons why newborn babies can recover from periods of oxygen deprivation that more mature humans cannot endure:

- In response to hypoxia, the baby conserves energy by shutting down the circulation to all but the most vital organs.
- After a latent period called primary apnoea, automatic, spinally generated gasping activity appears.
- While at the same time, the newborn baby's heart can utilise glycogen as an alternative fuel which allows it to provide an adequate circulation in the face of profound hypoxia and considerable biochemical disturbance for a reasonably long time. This circulatory resilience is a feature of all mammals at birth.

My key take-home messages from this chapter are:

The process of resuscitation at birth

In this chapter

Preparation for newborn resuscitation

After delivery
- Initial assessment and cord management
- Beginning resuscitation – thermal care, airway management and inflating (aerating) the lungs
- What to do if there is a response
- What to do if there is no response

Teamwork, leadership and communication

The learning outcomes will enable you to:

Understand how the preceding chapter on physiology relates to clinical practice

Recognise the importance of preparation

Recognise the baby who requires support or resuscitation

Use the NLS approach to resuscitate those few babies needing more than just gentle stimulation or support

Introduction

Resuscitation is likely to be rapidly successful if started before the baby has become so hypoxic that all potential for respiratory activity has vanished.[124] Babies in primary apnoea can usually resuscitate themselves if they have a clear airway and are kept warm. This ability to 'self-resuscitate' is why, in the past, a number of unusual methods of resuscitation were promoted even though we now know them to be ineffective and, in some cases, potentially harmful.

It is not possible, during the initial assessment, to determine whether the apnoeic newborn baby is in primary or secondary apnoea; this will only become apparent retrospectively as the baby is resuscitated. A structured, stepwise approach to management needs to be applied that will work in either situation. This starts with thermal care, assessment and considering optimal umbilical cord management then proceeds as far as necessary down the following simplified algorithm:

Dry and cover the baby
Assess the situation and consider umbilical cord management
A Airway
B Breathing (initial inflation breaths, then ventilation breaths)
C Circulation (chest compressions)
D (Drugs)

An overview of resuscitation

Dry and cover the baby

Always start by drying and covering the baby to prevent it from getting cold. A wet baby rapidly loses heat, and a small baby can quickly become dangerously hypothermic.[24] Babies subjected to cold stress in the period immediately after birth have a lower arterial oxygen tension and a worse metabolic acidosis,[25] and there is evidence in animals that hypoxia, acidosis and hypothermia all tend to inhibit surfactant production.[27] In very low birthweight babies, for each 1°C drop in body temperature below 36.5°C, the baseline mortality increases by 28%.[29]

Unless immediate resuscitative measures are required for mother or baby which cannot be done with the umbilical cord intact, the baby can remain attached to the placenta during initial assessment. The benefits of delayed umbilical cord clamping are covered in Chapter 6.

> Take measures to maintain a baby's temperature in the normal range – avoid both hypothermia and hyperthermia

Assessment and intervention

The assessment follows a logical order; during delivery and initial handling knowledge is gained on the appearance (colour) of the baby and its tone. Whilst instituting initial thermal care, observation of the chest permits an assessment of breathing. The heart rate must be actively determined, and this is best done at this stage by listening to the chest with a stethoscope. Your observations and the resuscitation measures that you then take should be accurately recorded.[125]

A = Airway

The majority of babies will start to breathe spontaneously as long as they have an open airway. If the airway is not open, air cannot be drawn into the lungs (Chapter 7). Babies in primary apnoea only require a clear airway in order to establish effective breathing – although as primary and terminal apnoea are not immediately distinguishable, inflation breaths are given.

B = Breathing

If the airway is clear and yet there is no effective breathing, it is necessary to fill the lungs with air, first by inflation breaths to clear lung fluid, and then ventilation breaths to maintain gas exchange (Chapter 7). In most cases, the circulation is still functioning, in which case the first sign of effective oxygen delivery to the heart will be a rise in the heart rate. Breathing efforts may then improve, at which point supportive ventilation might be discontinued. However, some babies, particularly those who are premature, may benefit from ongoing support through the use of continuous positive airway pressure (CPAP).

If the heart rate does not improve the most likely cause is failure to inflate the lungs and you should then check whether the lungs really have been inflated by checking for chest movement. Always ensure 30 s of adequate ventilation before proceeding to chest compressions. Starting inspired oxygen levels are shown in Table 5.1.

Table 5.1   Recommended initial oxygen concentrations in preterm babies

Gestation	Starting concentration of oxygen
> 32 weeks	Air
28+0 – 32+0 weeks	21–30%
< 28+0 weeks	30%

Titrate oxygen given to pre-ductal saturation targets (Table 5.2). Do not give supplemental oxygen if saturations are > 95%. If the heart rate is not responding despite effective ventilation supplemental oxygen is often used and if giving chest compressions increase to 100% oxygen.

Table 5.2   Acceptable right arm oxygen saturations after birth

Time from birth	Acceptable (25th centile) right arm oxygen saturations
2 min	65%
5 min	85%
10 min	90%

C = Circulation

Where the heart rate is very slow (less than 60 min[-1]) and there is no rise in heart rate despite lung inflation and adequate ventilation, as judged by visible chest movement for 30 s, then the circulation may need assistance using chest compressions (Chapter 8). If correctly performed, this will bring blood from the lungs to the heart. Provided the lungs have been aerated before chest compressions start, the blood that returns to the heart will be oxygenated and this will usually allow the heart to respond with an increase in heart rate.

D = Drugs

In a minority of babies, there may be no response despite good lung aeration, ventilation and effective chest compressions. This may be because of prolonged hypoxia with accumulation of lactic acid and/or exhaustion of the limited glycogen stores in the heart muscle. In this situation, stimulation of the myocardium and improvement of coronary artery perfusion (with adrenaline), the provision of energy (with glucose) and reversal of the acidosis within the heart (with sodium bicarbonate) may be successful (Chapter 8). If these drugs are used then venous access, usually via an umbilical venous catheter, will be necessary (Appendix 2). Adrenaline doses should be repeated every 3–5 minutes whilst CPR is ongoing.

Newborn life support

(Antenatal counselling)
Team briefing and equipment check

Birth
Delay cord clamping if possible

Start clock / note time
Dry / wrap, stimulate, keep warm

Assess
Colour, tone, breathing, heart rate

Ensure an open airway
Preterm: consider CPAP

If gasping / not breathing
- **Give 5 inflations (30 cm H_2O) – start in air**
- Apply PEEP 5–6 cm H_2O, if possible
- Apply SpO_2 +/- ECG

Reassess
If no increase in heart rate, look for chest movement

If the chest is not moving
- Check mask, head and jaw position
- 2 person support
- Consider suction, laryngeal mask/tracheal tube
- Repeat inflation breaths
- Consider increasing the inflation pressure

Reassess
If no increase in heart rate, look for chest movement

Once chest is moving continue ventilation breaths

If heart rate is not detectable or < 60 min^{-1}
after 30 seconds of ventilation
- Synchronise 3 chest compressions to 1 ventilation
- Increase oxygen to 100%
- Consider intubation if not already done or laryngeal mask if not possible

Reassess heart rate and chest movement
every 30 seconds

If the heart rate remains not detectable or < 60 min^{-1}
- **Vascular access and drugs**
- Consider other factors e.g. pneumothorax, hypovolaemia, congenital abormality

Update parents and debrief team
Complete records

Preterm
< 32 weeks

Place undried in plastic wrap + radiant heat

Inspired oxygen
28–31 weeks 21–30%
< 28 weeks 30%

If giving inflations, start with 25 cm H_2O

Acceptable pre-ductal SpO_2	
2 min	65%
5 min	85%
10 min	90%

TITRATE OXYGEN TO ACHIEVE TARGET SATURATIONS

APPROX 60 SECONDS

MAINTAIN TEMPERATURE

AT ALL TIMES ASK "IS HELP NEEDED"

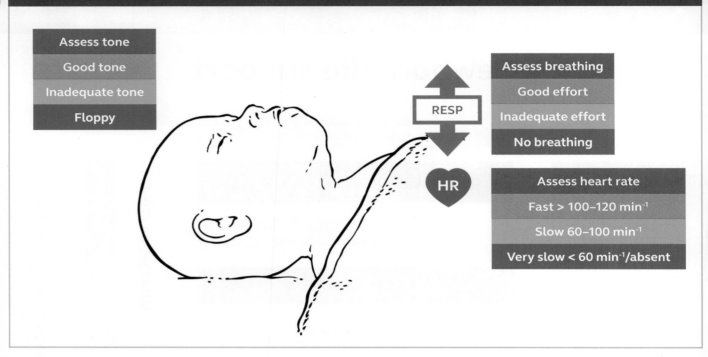

Figure 5.2   How the initial assessment can direct your interventions

Assess tone
Good tone
Inadequate tone
Floppy

RESP

Assess breathing
Good effort
Inadequate effort
No breathing

HR

Assess heart rate
Fast > 100–120 min^{-1}
Slow 60–100 min^{-1}
Very slow < 60 min^{-1}/absent

Timing of resuscitation events

There are no standard times by which certain events must be achieved, only that you should progress stepwise down the algorithm in a timely manner. Much will depend on the availability of help and equipment. In most cases, you should aim to complete your assessment and open the airway ready to begin inflation breaths by about 60 s after birth. A retrospective review of resuscitation events in babies who required full resuscitation showed these occurred at the following times in real-life (Table 5.3).[13]

Table 5.3   Real-life timing of key events during full resuscitation[13]

Key event	Median postnatal age
Chest movement achieved	1.0 min
Paediatric/neonatal team arrived	1.5 min
Chest compressions commenced	2.0 min
Central venous access obtained	9.0 min
First dose of adrenaline	10.0 min
First dose of bicarbonate	12.0 min

Preparation for resuscitation

The need for resuscitation of the newborn baby cannot always be predicted. Therefore, at every birth, no matter how 'low risk' the situation appears, the birth attendants must be prepared to resuscitate the newborn baby and know who and how to summon if further help is required. Certain situations (e.g. prematurity) are more likely to mean a baby needs assistance. Preparation and planning are covered in Chapter 6.

In any situation always ask:

1. **Do you need help?**

   At all times consider whether more help is required and if so, ensure it is summoned. Senior support may be needed, especially for preterm babies (Chapter 9). More staff may be needed for twins, especially if born by caesarean section; or if intra-partum monitoring suggests that the baby may have been severely compromised (e.g. a prolonged fetal bradycardia). When calling for help be clear who you need and where they need to come (Chapter 13).

2. **Is transport required?**

   If the baby is likely to be very small or preterm, consider whether you will transfer the baby on the resuscitaire or whether you will need to arrange to have a portable incubator and air/oxygen nearby for transfer. In the home, an ambulance may need to be called.

   Do you need help?

   Always ask for help if you expect or encounter any difficulty.

Preparation can often prevent difficulties. If you are attending a birth at home there can be a considerable delay between asking for help and receiving it. It is better to have help arrive and not need it than to find you really need help which has not yet been summoned.

After delivery

Drying and assessing the baby

- Start the clock or note the time of birth.
- Attend the baby with a warm, dry towel; consider cord management.
- Dry the baby promptly and effectively. Remove the wet towel and wrap in a fresh dry warm towel. (For very small or significantly preterm babies it is better to place the wet baby in a polythene bag or wrap – and place under a radiant heater). Cover the head with a hat or towel.
- During this period, it is possible to assess the baby and decide whether any intervention is going to be needed. For apparently well babies there is no need to rush to clamp the cord. Unless the baby is clearly in need of immediate resuscitation, wait for at least 60 s from the complete delivery of the baby before clamping the cord. Keep the baby warm during this time.

A non-crying baby may indicate that they require assistance.[4] If the baby is thought to need assistance then this becomes the priority. In order to provide assistance the baby may need to be moved; this, in turn, may require clamping and cutting the cord. If the baby is limp or very pale, has a very slow heart rate (less than 60 min⁻¹) or is making no effort to breathe, transfer the baby to the resuscitation area (Figure 5.2).

Stimulation

The process of delivery will often stimulate the baby, as will the subsequent handling and drying.[126] This is usually sufficient; avoid more aggressive methods of stimulation. Methods of tactile stimulation vary widely, for example, rubbing the soles of the feet, their back, or their chest; the optimal method remains unknown.[15,16] The benefits seem to be greater in preterm babies than in term babies.[17]

Initial assessment

The initial assessment is a clinical one and usually undertaken without the use of monitors. You need to assess the baby's:

colour

tone

breathing

heart rate

Colour

Colour does not appear in the algorithm (Figure 5.1) because it is not as good a means of assessing oxygenation, nor is it a reliable means of assessing how this is improving during resuscitation, as was often previously thought.[127] However, it is mentioned here because it is still thought to be useful for assessing the initial condition of the baby at birth. Babies in difficulty because of acidosis or serious blood loss will appear very pale at birth whereas the more usual colour is blue. Very pale babies who remain pale after resuscitation may be hypovolaemic as well as acidotic.

Tone

Babies born well-flexed and with good tone are usually fine. A baby who is very floppy is unconscious and in significant difficulties. The tone of a baby is often clear from its posture but can also be rapidly assessed by handling the baby.

Breathing

Breathing usually starts spontaneously within a minute of birth and whilst apnoea on assessment should prompt action it is important to realise that some perfectly healthy babies can take up to three minutes to start breathing after birth.[38] This does not mean that you should simply leave the baby until they start to breathe; instead you should facilitate delayed cord clamping, stimulate the baby and continue to assess them. The baby may show normal regular breaths, irregular breaths, gasping (sometimes interspersed amongst more normal breaths), or breathing may be absent (apnoea). The baby who does not cry after birth might be apnoeic or may be breathing; whilst the apnoeic group clearly need attention, the latter group also require careful and ongoing assessment.[4]

Gasping breaths are usually accompanied by subcostal, intercostal and sternal recession but recession (consisting of a drawing in of the skin between, or under the ribs, or of the sternum itself) is also occasionally seen with regular breathing, suggesting increased work of breathing perhaps due to partial obstruction of the airway or stiff lungs in premature babies.[128]

Heart rate

In most healthy term and well preterm babies, the heart rate is usually greater than 100 min⁻¹ by 2 minutes of age,[38] although it can temporarily decrease after immediate cord clamping before recovering. This decrease in heart rate is not seen with delayed cord clamping.

Assessing the heart rate can be done in several ways (Table 5.4).

Table 5.4 Methods of assessing the heart rate during resuscitation. These methods are displayed in the order that they are likely to be used.

Using a stethoscope
When first assessing the heart rate, use a stethoscope. It is usually clear whether the heart rate is very slow (less than 60 min⁻¹), slow (60–100 min⁻¹) or fast (more than 100 min⁻¹). It is not necessary to count it with complete accuracy. Although the cardiac impulse may often be felt at the umbilicus or the apex it cannot always be felt. Consequently, the rate judged by cord pulsation, if slow, may not reflect the true heart rate.[39]
Pulse oximetry
A pulse oximeter allows an accurate assessment of heart rate and oxygen saturation. Attempting to judge oxygenation by assessing skin colour is unreliable[127] but it is still worth noting the baby's colour at birth as well as whether, when and how it changes.
ECG monitoring
This has been demonstrated to rapidly and accurately determine the heart rate at birth.[129] A reliable ECG signal can be obtained more quickly than a pulse oximetry signal, however it only registers the electrical heart beat (i.e. there is an electrical signal), not whether there is any effective cardiac output.[130]

A pulse oximeter will give accurate assessment of heart rate and oxygen saturation in less than 15 s of application;[131,132] this will typically be about 90 s after birth.[133] Saturation levels in healthy babies in the first few minutes of life may be considerably lower than at other times.[134] In babies at birth, the arterial oxygen saturation may be different depending on whether it is measured in areas supplied by blood leaving the aorta before or after the entry of the arterial duct (i.e. whether they are pre-ductal or post-ductal measurements). Measurements taken in the right arm are pre-ductal whereas measurements from other limbs will be post-ductal. Pre-ductal saturations represent the oxygen going to the brain, for this reason saturations should be measured in the right arm.

Values in Table 5.2 are based on those from healthy newborn babies of all gestations who received neither resuscitation nor additional oxygen. The data came from 308 term babies, 121 babies between 32 and 36 weeks gestation and 39 babies under 32 weeks gestation.[134]

The saturation levels listed in Table 5.2 are deemed 'acceptable' in the sense that babies exhibiting these levels probably do not need any supplemental oxygen. However, babies whose saturation levels are significantly lower might warrant careful supplementation. Babies with oxygen saturations of 95% or more do not need added oxygen (or if they are receiving oxygen this needs to be reduced).

A pulse oximeter can be very helpful in giving an accurate readout of heart rate and also has the advantage of giving information on oxygen saturation. If you don't have a pulse oximeter or an ECG, a stethoscope is the most reliable means of monitoring heart rate.

If a baby has reasonable tone, appears well and is making some respiratory effort, despite a slow heart rate, then it is reasonable to wait a minute or so, whilst both stimulating it and ensuring that the head is appropriately positioned to open the airway.

If the baby has a good heart rate and is making good respiratory effort, then no further help is required. Once wrapped, this baby should be given to the mother and skin-to-skin contact encouraged.

Airway, breathing, circulation (and drugs)

These steps must be tackled in this order (Figure 5.1). It will not be possible to aerate the lungs without an open airway. Blood cannot be oxygenated unless air is delivered to the lungs. Chest compressions are pointless without oxygenated blood to move from the lungs to the heart.

Airway opening manoeuvres

If a baby is not breathing adequately, or is gasping, then the first step is to open the airway. The airway may be obstructed if the neck is either too flexed or too extended or – in a floppy baby on its back – if the tongue falls back into the airway due to loss of pharyngeal tone (Chapter 7). These mechanisms are more likely to be the cause of an airway problem than any mechanical obstruction from blood, thick mucus, or lumps of vernix or meconium.

After opening the airway and stimulation some babies start to make satisfactory breathing efforts in which case continue to support the airway and observe. Reassess the heart rate to ensure this is satisfactory. No other action may be required.

Meconium

Screaming babies	Have an open airway
Floppy babies	Begin the standard A, B, C approach.
	Consider airway suction if airway opening manoeuvres do not result in chest movement during inflation breaths.

Most babies born through meconium-stained liquor have not inhaled any particulate material into the lower respiratory tract. If they have not done so as a result of anoxic gasping before birth, they will only very rarely do so at birth.[135] Suction of the baby's airways on the perineum or routine suction after delivery are not recommended. In a bradycardic baby, the emphasis must be to inflate the lungs within the first minute after birth and this should not be delayed. Do not inspect the oropharynx or suction the trachea until you have attempted, and been unable to inflate the chest despite standard airway opening manoeuvres. There is no evidence to support routine tracheal suctioning in this situation.[136] If you fail to inflate the lungs and you strongly suspect airway obstruction, inspect the airway under direct vision.

Inflation breaths

In order to clear lung fluid in an unresponsive baby, positive pressure inflations with a 2–3 s inspiration time are required (Chapter 6). For a term baby, start at pressures of about 30 cm water[137] with inflation times sustained for 2–3 s.[138] Five such 'inflation breaths' should be sufficient to aerate the lung. Significantly preterm babies (32 weeks and below) may respond to a lower initial inflation pressure of 25 cm water (Chapter 9).[139,140] In all babies of ≥ 32 weeks gestation, it is recommended to start resuscitation with air (21% oxygen); for babies between 28 and 32 weeks, start with 21–30% oxygen and for babies < 28 weeks gestation start with 30% oxygen.

> Having given five inflation breaths – reassess to see if the baby has responded.
>
> **Reassess – has the heart rate improved?**

Heart rate is increasing

If inflation breaths have aerated the lungs, you would expect the heart rate to increase within 5–10 s.[141] This is one of the first signs that the baby is responding. If the heart rate is increasing rapidly, you can assume that you have successfully aerated the lungs. You then proceed as follows:

Ventilation support

Following inflation breaths, the baby may start breathing spontaneously. If this does not occur, gently ventilate the lungs at about 30 breaths min[-1] until the baby starts to breathe. If your ventilation is adequate, the heart rate will remain above 100 beats min[-1]. If it falls below this, it suggests that your ventilation is inadequate. Recheck the airway position and ventilation technique. Pressures of ~25 cm water and inspiratory times of about 1 s are usually adequate for ventilation once the lungs have been inflated. In preterm babies start with a pressure of 25 cm water. If chest movement is generous, then pressures can be reduced.

Reassess – is there spontaneous breathing?

With continued support, breathing efforts will usually return. The manner in which they return is important. If the first efforts are gasping in nature, this would suggest that the baby may have been in terminal apnoea. It is important to record the sequence and timing of events. If the heart rate is satisfactory but no spontaneous breathing returns, then you might consider other factors such as sedation, neurological issues or intrathoracic pathology. Remember, it is possible to render a healthy baby apnoeic by lowering the $PaCO_2$ with hyperventilation.

Heart rate is not increasing

If the heart rate is not responding the most likely reason is that you have failed to aerate the lungs. Go back and check airway-opening manoeuvres and repeat the inflation breaths.

This is the time to consider using two-person airway support and other airway manoeuvres (Chapter 7).

Reassess – is there chest movement?

In the absence of a heart rate response, seeing the chest move as you give inflation breaths is the only way to judge successful aeration of the lungs. Listening for breath sounds with a stethoscope can be misleading because of transmitted upper airway sounds. Chest movement may only start to occur after the first few (two or three) effective inflation breaths. Check for chest movement as you give a further set of inflation breaths. Once you have confirmed chest movement, ventilate for 30 s and then reassess.

Reassess – is the heart rate satisfactory?

If the heart rate remains slow or absent, despite adequate ventilation for 30 s as shown by chest movement, then you need to give chest compressions (Chapter 8). Chest compressions should help to move oxygenated blood from the lungs to the heart and coronary arteries. The blood you move can only be oxygenated if the lungs have air in them. At this point it is recommended that you increase the inspired oxygen to 100%.

Reassess – has the heart rate improved?

It is usually only necessary to continue chest compressions for about 20–30 s before the heart responds with an increase in heart rate.[12]

Consider drugs

If the baby has been subjected to severe hypoxic stress, these simple measures may not be enough to produce an increase in heart rate. In this situation it may be necessary to use drugs to stimulate the heart. The venous access necessary to give these drugs is most easily achieved using an umbilical venous catheter, although intraosseous access is an alternative. Adrenaline doses should be repeated every 3–5 minutes whilst CPR is ongoing.

Reassess – has the heart rate improved?

If the heart rate is still not improving (see Chapter 8), consider other factors such as hypovolaemia, tension pneumothorax, diaphragmatic hernia or, rarely, complete heart block.

Reassess – should resuscitation attempts continue?

If there was no detectable heart rate at birth and still none by ten minutes of age, the attending team should review the clinical factors such as gestation of the baby, the quality and effectiveness of resuscitation, the availability of therapeutic hypothermia and the views of the team regarding the continuation of resuscitation. Any problems with resuscitation techniques should be addressed with special consideration given to securing the airway with either a laryngeal mask or by intubation if this has not already occurred. Parents should be updated and made aware of the situation.

If the heart rate of a term baby remains undetectable for more than 20 min after birth despite resuscitation and the exclusion of reversible causes, then it may be appropriate to stop resuscitation (see Chapter 11). In the preterm baby this point may be reached earlier.

If, after extensive resuscitation, there is a detectable but slow heart rate the prognosis may also be very poor. In this case the decision to cease resuscitation is less clear and it may be appropriate to take the baby to the intensive care unit where additional facilities for monitoring and intervention exist.

Palliative (comfort-focused) care should be used whenever life sustaining treatment is withheld or withdrawn.

Teamwork, leadership and communication

In the majority of cases, simple resuscitative measures result in a speedy recovery, and additional help is not required. In a minority of cases, additional help is required, and in order to be effective any intervention needs the right people to be working together in the right place at the right time, and with the right equipment. How this is achieved is discussed in Chapters 6 and 13.

In an emergency, structured communication helps. Communication problems are a factor in up to 80% of adverse incidents or near miss reports in hospitals. This failure of communication can easily occur during a newborn emergency. A person calling for help may fail to communicate the seriousness of the situation, or convey the information in a way that does not ensure that the recipient appreciates the urgency of the situation. A well-structured process that is simple, reliable and dependable will enable the caller to convey the important facts, the degree of urgency and allow the recipient to plan ahead.

Use of the acronym, SBAR (Situation, Background, Assessment, Recommendation) (Table 5.5) is now widely accepted across the health service and can be helpful in planning effective, timely communication between individuals from different clinical backgrounds and hierarchies.

Table 5.5   SBAR (Situation, Background, Assessment, Recommendation)

SBAR	Content	Example A	Example B
Situation	• Introduce yourself and check you are speaking to the correct person. • Identify the patient you are calling about (who and where). • State what you need.	*I am the senior midwife on the labour ward.* *I am calling about Ms Smith.* *There is cord prolapse and we are proceeding to immediate section.*	*I am the senior midwife on the labour ward.* *I am calling about baby Smith in room five.* *The baby is grunting at one hour of age.*
Background	Important features of pregnancy and delivery. Term or preterm. Condition at birth and response to any resuscitation.	*Pregnancy has been normal.* *This is a term labour that was normal until the membranes ruptured five minutes ago.* *The umbilical cord has prolapsed.*	*Pregnancy has been normal.* *Delivery was by elective section for breech at 38 weeks.* *The baby was in good condition at birth and did not need resuscitation, but has been grunting since 10 minutes of age.*
Assessment	Undelivered mother • Progression of labour, CTG findings. Baby • colour, tone, breathing, heart rate.	*The cord is in the vagina.* *It is still pulsating.*	*Baby is pink in air,* *HR is > 100, tone is normal,* *RR is 60 per minute with grunting.*
Recommendation	• What by when?	*Please attend theatre one immediately.* *Please alert your seniors.*	*I am not too concerned, but I would like you to review the baby within 30 minutes.*

05: Summary learning

The approach to newborn resuscitation follows a standard algorithm:

- dry and cover the baby
- assess the situation and consider umbilical cord management
- airway
- breathing (initial inflation breaths, then ventilation breaths)
- chest compressions
- (drugs).

Preparation is an essential component of successful resuscitation.

Most babies respond quickly to simple basic life support.

More complicated and prolonged resuscitation requires teamwork, leadership and effective communication.

My key take-home messages from this chapter are:

Anticipation, preparation and umbilical cord management

Anticipation and preparation for delivery, transition and resuscitation

For many deliveries, a risk assessment will allow planning for the likelihood of a baby needing support or intervention after birth and ensures appropriate people and equipment are available. Anticipating delivery room resuscitation enables the team to plan the care of the baby and sometimes allows time to counsel the family prior to delivery. In some situations, this may involve the antenatal transfer of the mother to a centre designated to provide an appropriate level of neonatal care. This is important because babies born extremely prematurely have better outcomes if they are born and cared for in centres with level 3 neonatal services, particularly those with high activity.[142-144] The same may be true of other high-risk fetal or neonatal conditions such as some cardiac or surgical condition or surgical problems which may require immediate support.[145]

Deliveries may be stratified into 'low-risk', 'moderate-risk', and 'high-risk' guiding the need for a resuscitation team presence at birth, even when transfer for specialist care is not warranted.[18,146,147] Remember that babies born from deliveries stratified as 'low-risk' may unexpectedly require assistance. Local guidelines indicating who should attend deliveries should be developed, based on current understanding of best practice and clinical audit, and should consider these risk factors (Table 6.1). The neonatal/paediatric team should ensure that they are part of any pre-surgery checklist when they are called to attend a caesarean section. The WHO Surgical Safety Checklist,[148] shown to improve patient safety as well as improving teamwork and communication, became a mandatory requirement for all NHS hospitals in England and Wales in 2009.

Table 6.1 Risk factors that may indicate the need for advanced resuscitation or additional steps to be taken at delivery. These may be identified before, or may become apparent during, labour.

Antepartum factors affecting the fetus	Prematurity < 37 weeks gestation	Fetal anaemia or isoimmunisation (including hydrops)
	Intrauterine growth restriction	Oligo- or polyhydramnios
	Multiple pregnancy	Serious congenital abnormalities
Maternal antenatal factors	Maternal sepsis and fever	High BMI
	Gestational diabetes	Short stature
	Pregnancy induced hypertension	Lack of antenatal steroids (preterm deliveries)
	Pre-eclampsia	
Intrapartum factors	Evidence of fetal compromise (e.g. non-reassuring CTG, pathological CTG)	Significant maternal haemorrhage
	Meconium-stained amniotic fluid	Caesarean section before 39 weeks
	Vaginal breech delivery	Emergency caesarean section
	Instrumental (i.e. forceps or vacuum) delivery	General anaesthesia

Antenatally diagnosed conditions and implications for resuscitation

In most instances, antenatal diagnosis allows for forward planning for the delivery of babies with congenital anomalies. However, nature (and the baby) may have other ideas, and the delivery may occur before the team can arrive or before the mother can be transferred to the tertiary centre. This section gives a brief overview of some of the more common anomalies (all of which are rare in themselves) and suggests how a person with basic newborn resuscitation knowledge and skills can support that baby until additional help arrives.

In most cases, the standard NLS approach can be used either unchanged or with some minor modifications.

Congenital heart disease

Most congenital heart disease does not, in the absence of hydrops, require additional support at birth. As the ductus arteriosus remains open, even those with complex, duct-dependent congenital heart anomalies can be managed using the standard NLS algorithm. Some congenital heart abnormalities mean that oxygen saturations will not reach normal levels and the baby will remain cyanosed. Call for senior support as soon as possible. Ongoing management of the congenital heart disease can take place once the baby is stabilised.

Intrathoracic masses

There are a number of intrathoracic congenital pathologies but few cause immediate problems at birth, and a standard NLS approach can be used. One important exception is a congenital diaphragmatic hernia which may cause respiratory compromise at birth. The birth of such babies should be discussed and planned so that an experienced resuscitation team is available as early intubation at birth is usually required.

Conditions that carry a high risk for neonatal airway obstruction

Airway obstruction may occur at any level of the airway and may be caused by external compression or intrinsic structural abnormalities. The fetus with known severe micrognathia or congenital abnormalities of the neck or airway may be at significant risk of airway obstruction at delivery. As before, the birth of any such babies would be planned to include the availability of an experienced resuscitation team, often in regional or supra-regional specialist centres.

Babies with micrognathia may be manageable using some of the airway techniques described in this manual (e.g. laryngeal mask, two handed jaw support, oro- or naso-pharyngeal airways, positioning – prone or side-lying) and these procedures should be attempted before resorting to more invasive measures.

Neural tube defects (including encephalocoele and myelomeningocele)

The breathing of babies with encephalocoele may be impaired because of airway obstruction or central apnoea. Although senior help should be called, they usually require no more than routine resuscitation measures and sometimes positioning on their side with appropriate airway and breathing assessment. Babies with myelomeningocele generally do not have respiratory problems, however, an associated hydrocephalus may cause the neck to be flexed and the airway to be compromised when in the supine position. In addition, steps should be taken to protect the exposed neural elements and prevent rupture of the membrane covering the defect; place the baby in a prone or side-lying position and cover the lesion with sterile saline-soaked gauze and a plastic wrap covering.

Abdominal wall defects (exomphalos and gastroschisis)

Thermoregulation and fluid loss are concerns here because the baby may lose heat through the exposed viscera and insensible fluid loss is significant. A sterile plastic bag is often placed over the lower extremities and trunk to the level of the nipple line.

If positive pressure ventilation is required, consider passing a nasogastric tube to minimise intestinal distension, and expedite elective tracheal intubation. If emergency vascular access is required, consider the intraosseous route, as umbilical venous catheterisation may be difficult or impossible.

Skeletal dysplasias

Effective antenatal communication between obstetrics, genetics, neonatal providers and the parents is essential. This enables as full an understanding as possible about the current status of the fetus, the most likely diagnosis and prognosis and may inform resuscitation decisions. Special consideration should be given to the possibility of pulmonary hypoplasia (where a higher pressure may be required) or bone fragility (where gentle handling is required). Chest compressions, if required, should not be withheld for fear that they may cause rib fractures.[149]

Renal anomalies

Renal anomalies are among the most frequently detected problems on antenatal screening. In the presence of normal liquor volumes, they do not usually present with additional problems requiring resuscitation. If the liquor volume is reduced or absent then the baby may have severe respiratory problems due to pulmonary hypoplasia (Potter's sequence); higher pressures may be required to inflate the lungs and the prognosis for such infants remains poor.[150]

Communication between obstetric, midwifery and newborn teams

Labour and delivery are almost unique in healthcare in that they result in two (or more) patients being cared for in the same room, by two or more teams of healthcare providers. Effective communication between the teams is essential for delivery of optimal care, yet national reports continue to highlight the lack of timely or effective communication.[151-154] The WHO Surgical Safety Checklist, or a variation of this, should be used for caesarean sections and should include the neonatal/paediatric team in the discussions.

Information that can inform the choice of neonatal personnel as well as decisions about umbilical cord management include:

- **How many babies are expected?** Each baby should have at least one trained provider and each baby may need its own resuscitaire and other equipment.
- **What is the gestational age?** Lower gestational age will increase the likelihood of need for stabilisation. More experienced providers should be present at these deliveries and ensure that there is appropriate equipment for the gestational age.
- **Is the amniotic fluid clear?** Meconium may indicate antenatal fetal distress, and hence the increased likelihood of needing resuscitation, including the possibility of airway obstruction if adequate ventilation is not achieved. Bloody fluid may indicate the possibility of haemorrhage, which is usually, but not always, maternal due to placental abruption.
- **Are there any additional risk factors?** The obstetric and midwifery team can provide information on other risk factors that may guide preparation and resuscitation (e.g. CTG abnormalities, medications used for maternal analgesia, etc.) These may prompt an additional call for help or for other team members.
- **What is the preferred management of the umbilical cord after delivery and facilitation of delayed cord clamping?** Management of the cord (see later in this chapter) requires well-planned interaction and communication between the clinical teams.

Communication with the parents before delivery

NICE guidelines provide recommendations for communicating with all mothers, including simple instructions on greetings, demeanour, establishing rapport, and maintaining a respectful and safe environment.[155] This meeting and discussion should cover aspects described in Table 6.2.[156] This may need to be adapted according to time available for such discussions. The discussion should be documented contemporaneously if there is sufficient time.

Table 6.2 Suggested contents for the consultation with parents when additional support for the newborn baby is anticipated

What is the clinical presentation and the facts or evidence needed to inform decision-making?	Before meeting the family obtain clinical information and consult with team members (+/- specialist services or neonatal centres) as required
	Consider evidence search for complex situations
What are the options for treatment for this presentation?	Share the case with relevant team members or referral units
How will you approach the mother and their support person or family?	Knock, if appropriate
	Clear introduction with your names and your roles
	Sit, if possible, and maintain a private, quiet environment
	Allow silence for thought and questions
How will you establish rapport and a two-way dialogue? (or "What do you need to know?")	Enquire about their circumstances
	What do they wish to know?
	What are their concerns?
	What is their decision-making style?
What do they need to know?	Tailor conversation to needs of parents and the specific situation
	Provide a balanced perspective of morbidities and mortality, and realistic treatment options
	This may include discussion on coping and adaptation to NICU and subsequent care
How do they react to the conversation?	Discuss goals, hopes, and fears
	Debrief and support with ongoing offer of consultation and NICU visit

Figure 6.1	A suggestion for a pre-brief checklist	

Team member introductions and allocation of roles	✓

Patient situation	
Relevant maternal/family history	
Diagnosis	
Gestational age	
Estimated weight (informed by fetal weight estimations or by average for gestation)	
Whether participating in any research studies and protocol to support that	
In cases with high mortality or morbidity, is there an agreed Anticipatory Care Pathway that outlines the parental wishes and expectations and/or limits of action?	

Anticipated stabilisation or resuscitation steps	
Management of the umbilical cord	
Thermal management (e.g. allocating role of temperature monitoring and control in a preterm delivery)	
Positioning considerations (e.g. spina bifida – prone or side-lying, abdominal wall defects – on their back with attention to the exposed bowel)	
Starting FiO_2 and pulse oximetry goals (see Chapter 7)	
Airway and breathing management plan	
Vascular access needs	

Equipment	
Check of standard equipment – is it all there, does it work?	
Any additional equipment required?	

Escalation procedure	
Who do we need to call for additional support if needed, and how?	
Are the people who might be called for support aware of the situation?	

Team brief and preparation for a resuscitation

It is important to have adequate personnel available at every birth; local guidelines may vary in regard to personnel availability. Every birth should be attended by at least one individual who is competent to provide the initial steps of newborn life support. This individual should only be responsible for the care of the newborn.[31] For deliveries with risk factors (Table 6.1), additional personnel should be present to provide neonatal resuscitation as needed.

For more complex situations where a team of personnel is required, assigning roles helps to ensure clarity, efficiency, and to avoid duplication. A pre-delivery briefing allows the resuscitation team to briefly to discuss the resuscitation plans before the birth. The team briefing, although no more than a few minutes, will ensure adequate preparation for the delivery and help to optimise key behavioural skills in neonatal resuscitation such as leadership, anticipation and planning, workload delegation, and use of available resources (Chapter 13). A pre-delivery briefing checklist may be helpful (Figure 6.1).

Umbilical cord clamping

The optimal time of cord clamping has been widely studied and delayed cord clamping (DCC) is safe and does not increase maternal adverse outcomes (e.g. post-partum haemorrhage). The terms 'delayed' and 'deferred' are often used interchangeably.

The preferred cord management options are:

1. At least 60 s of DCC unless it would prevent immediate resuscitation measures that are felt to be necessary

2. If resuscitation is required and at least 60 s of DCC is not practical, then cord milking (intact or cut cord) is an option in babies > 28 weeks gestation. Cord milking should not be practised in babies born earlier than 28 weeks gestation

3. In some cases, immediate cord clamping may be needed

Cord management requires planning and communication between the teams involved and with the parents.

The concept that the umbilical cord should not be clamped immediately is termed 'delayed' cord clamping (DCC). Unfortunately, this implies that 'immediate' cord clamping (ICC) is the normal or natural timing for cord clamping; physiological data (Chapter 4) and history would suggest otherwise.

The history of umbilical cord clamping

In 'primitive' human cultures, the cord is not cut until after the placenta has been delivered, sometimes hours later.[157] The earliest recorded evidence of interest in when the umbilical cord should be tied or clamped extends back centuries, at least to ancient Greece, where Aristotle observed that:

"Frequently the child appears to be born dead, when it is feeble and when, before the tying of the cord, a flux of blood occurs into the cord and adjacent parts...and at once the baby, who had previously been as if drained of blood, comes to life again."[158]

It is unclear when the practice of cutting the cord before placental delivery (i.e. ICC) started but evidence suggests it was emerging in the 17th and 18th centuries ostensibly to reduce maternal blood loss, the mess on the bed and to allow identification of cord lengthening.

Not everyone was convinced of its value, Charles White argued that it had 'nothing to plead in its favour but custom'.[159] A view shared by William Smellie (1697-1763) in his treatise on the theory and practice of midwifery when he wrote of the benefits of waiting until the infant cried before clamping the cord and observed how:

"if the air does not immediately rush into the lungs, and the circulation continues between [the baby] and the placenta, the operation of tying and cutting must be delayed, and everything tried to stimulate and sometimes to give pain... Whatever augments the circulating force, promotes respiration; and as this increases, the circulation grows stronger, so that they mutually assist each other."[160]

A cord clamp (like those used today) was invented in 1899, there was, however, no intention that it would lead to ICC and its inventor Edward Magennis advised clamping of the cord using his device "when it has ceased to pulsate".[161]

Several other practices contributed to a rise in early cord clamping; in the 1930s 'placental blood banks' were established in some countries.[162,163] The 'Hinchingbrooke' trial[164] saw the triad of uterotonic administration, ICC and controlled cord traction become established in the modern (active) management of the third stage of labour. Increasing delivery by caesarean section may also have inadvertently contributed to the acceptance of ICC; in the 1950s, only 3% of births in England were by caesarean section; by the beginning of the 21st century this had risen to 21%.[165] One survey suggested that avoiding delays in neonatal resuscitation was widely held as 'a reason to clamp the cord immediately'.[166]

None of the various reasons for early cord clamping have been demonstrated to be beneficial for the baby. There has been ongoing interest in the benefits of DCC in all settings and it is the results of this and the undertaking of properly conducted randomised controlled trials that are starting to inform practice.

Undertaking delayed cord clamping

The management of the umbilical cord begins before delivery with, if time permits, a discussion with the parents regarding the process of delayed cord clamping. If this is not the first baby that the mother has had, then delayed cord clamping (DCC) may be a novel experience if ICC was part of the mother's prior expectations.[167,168]

Overall, no increases in adverse maternal outcomes were reported (i.e. post-partum haemorrhage, use of uterotonics, etc.) or adverse neonatal outcomes (i.e. requirements for phototherapy in hyperbilirubinaemia, the incidence of necrotising enterocolitis, severe intraventricular haemorrhage, etc.). Benefits of cord clamping are shown in Tables 6.3 and 6.4.

Table 6.3 **Benefits of delayed versus immediate cord clamping in term infants** (adapted from the meta-analysis by Gomersall et al[169])

Parameter
Avoidance of bradycardia seen after ICC and the abrupt cardiovascular changes associated with that
Improved early haematological indices: • peak haemoglobin in first 24-hours
Improved iron stores in infancy

Table 6.4 **Benefits of delayed versus immediate cord clamping in preterm infants born before 34 weeks gestation** (adapted from the meta-analysis by Seidler et al[170])

Parameter
Improved survival
Improved early haematological indices: • peak haemoglobin in first 24-hours   • peak haematocrit in first 24-hours   • peak haematocrit at 7 days
Improved cardiovascular stability in first 24-hours   • less use of inotropic support   • higher mean blood pressure values
Blood transfusion requirements: • lower requirements for any blood transfusion   • lower total number of blood transfusions

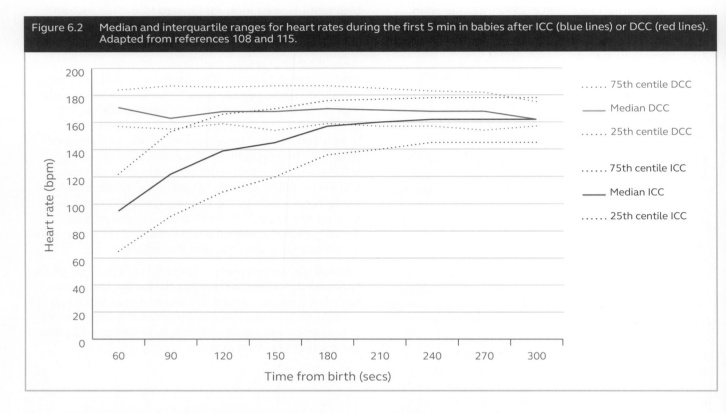

Figure 6.2 Median and interquartile ranges for heart rates during the first 5 min in babies after ICC (blue lines) or DCC (red lines). Adapted from references 108 and 115.

Some of the benefit is probably due to the increased circulating blood volume after DCC, but the heart rate is more stable when transitioning if DCC is used compared to ICC. Figure 6.2 shows composite data from two studies of changes in heart rate in the first few minutes after birth. Median heart rates from babies in the study by Dawson and colleagues[108] who had no interventions other than ICC are shown in blue. These contrast with data from babies (red lines) in the study reported by Blank and colleagues[115] when cord clamping was delayed for at least 2 min; these babies were less likely to have a bradycardia immediately after birth. The physiology behind this is discussed in Chapter 4.

There is no universally accepted definition of DCC, only that it does not occur immediately after the baby is born. Recent systematic reviews and meta-analyses have defined early or immediate cord clamping (ICC) clamping within 30 s of birth: with delayed cord clamping as being clamping at a time longer than 30 s.[169] A further definition, but for which there are fewer clinical data, is one based on physiological parameters (such as when cord pulsation has ceased or breathing has been initiated).

The recommended option is to delay cord clamping for at least 60 s.

This could be longer if the baby's temperature can be maintained and might even extend to after the baby's first breaths. Alternatives, for when DCC is not possible, include intact cord milking and cut cord milking. Both offer advantages for the baby over ICC, but not to the same extent as DCC.[169] Planning to undertake DCC as part of the stabilisation process also requires planning and should feature in the pre-delivery multi-disciplinary team brief.[171]

In a healthy baby, DCC can simply occur during drying and gentle stimulation; the baby is then placed skin-to-skin on the mother's abdomen and covered to ensure they remain warm. Assessment of the baby's colour, tone, breathing and heart rate can be undertaken during this period which will probably take about 30 s. The baby who is crying needs no further support.

Although 60 s after delivery is recommended as a minimum, there is some suggestion that a longer delay may be better,[170] perhaps because it allows for a smoother physiological transition between fetal and infant respiration (Chapter 4).

The non-crying baby should be assessed more closely; close observation and intervention may be needed.[4] Some parts of the standard algorithm, for example, opening the airway, can be undertaken whilst the baby remains skin-to-skin; but it may be necessary to offer additional support which realistically can only be done on a resuscitaire. The team must then make a choice whether to clamp the cord and take the baby to the resuscitaire, or whether leave the cord unclamped and to bring a resuscitaire to the baby. Local policy and facilities will probably dictate which route is followed.

Resuscitation whilst undertaking DCC has been shown to be feasible utilising a standard mobile resuscitaire or a mother-side resuscitaire[172] with the latter having being designed especially for this approach. Resuscitation should then follow the standard NLS approach. Whilst animal studies suggest that DCC during resuscitation from a hypoxic induced asphyxia insult can be protective,[173] the evidence of long-term benefit in humans is not yet clear. Some short-term outcome data do suggest benefit with shorter times to spontaneous breathing and higher Apgar scores at one, five and ten minutes in one randomised controlled trial of non-breathing term infants randomised to DCC.[174]

There are, as yet, few long-term outcome data to inform any firm recommendation about resuscitation during DCC. The picture is complicated by the multiple underlying causes for intrapartum asphyxia and include placenta abruption and a number of other situations where DCC may not be advisable (Table 6.5). In these cases, the cord must either be clamped immediately or consideration given to cord milking, where possible.

Table 6.5 Situations where delayed cord clamping may not be advisable

Cases with interruption of the placental blood flow/oxygenation:
• maternal haemorrhage • maternal seizure or cardiac arrest • placenta abruption • vasa praevia • cord avulsion
Fetal hydrops due to any underlying cause
Twin-to-twin transfusion syndrome

Umbilical cord milking

Umbilical cord milking has not been studied as widely as DCC but is recommended as an option for babies > 28 weeks when DCC is not possible.

There are two types of cord milking:

1. **Umbilical cord milking with an intact cord**

   In this procedure the umbilical cord is gently grasped as far away from the baby as possible, that hand then gently milks the cord towards the baby, usually 3–5 times. This can result in a faster blood flow than occurs with passive blood return (which is driven by the uterine contractions). During 3–5 of these milkings, a term infant may receive about 50 mL of blood.[175] After milking the cord is clamped and cut and the baby is taken to the resuscitaire.[176]

2. **Umbilical cord milking from a length of cut cord**

   In this procedure the cord is clamped as far away from the baby as possible. In a term baby this gives about 25 cm of cord (less in a preterm baby where cords are usually shorter). The baby is taken to the resuscitaire immediately and milking, undertaken in a similar manner to that described above, occurs during resuscitation.[177]

In term and near-term babies, meta-analysis comparing different cord milking strategies with ICC or DCC included few studies and reported few outcomes, therefore no clear differences in outcomes were seen.[169] More studies allowed for a few more comparisons in preterm infants; these are summarised in Table 6.6.

The concerns regarding an excess of intraventricular haemorrhage in very preterm infants appears real; animal studies of cord milking demonstrate that this procedure can cause marked haemodynamic fluctuations in arterial blood pressure and cerebral blood flow.[179] These are thought to be injurious to the immature cerebral circulation. **For this reason, cord milking should not be undertaken in infants < 28 weeks gestation.**

Table 6.6 Summary of clinical outcomes from the meta-analyses of trials in preterm infants comparing different cord care strategies (adapted from Seidler et al[170]).

Comparison	Statistically significant outcomes and comments
Immediate cord clamping (ICC) versus intact cord milking	Intact cord milking improves early haematological indices (peak haemoglobin and peak haematocrit) less use of inotropes on day 1 and fewer transfusions. Few long-term outcomes reported and none reached statistical or clinical significance.
DCC versus cut cord milking	No studies were identified for inclusion in the meta-analysis.
DCC versus intact cord milking	Intact cord milking appeared to offer the same benefits as DCC, however, of some concern was that one large study of intact cord milking versus DCC was terminated early when analysis demonstrated a significant excess of severe intraventricular haemorrhage in those infants born before 28 weeks allocated to the intact cord milking arm.[178]
ICC versus cut cord milking	Insufficient data to show any improved outcomes in either arm (only one small study included in the meta-analysis).*
* Outcome measures included neonatal survival, survival to discharge, complications of prematurity (including intraventricular haemorrhage, necrotising enterocolitis).	

06: Summary learning

Risk assessment, anticipation and preparation can help ensure the right support is available in a timely fashion at all deliveries; the higher the anticipated risk the more likely a team of people or senior clinicians are required.

A pre-delivery team brief is extremely helpful in higher risk and complex cases.

Some antenatally diagnosed conditions have implications for transition and resuscitation. Early notice of these can ensure antenatal transfer to a suitable place of delivery. Most conditions can be managed using the standard NLS approach.

Communication between team members, between teams and with parents is paramount.

Cord management, in particular, requires planning and communication between the teams involved and with the parents.

We recommend at least 60 s of DCC unless it would prevent resuscitation. If this is not practical alternatives are:

- Cord milking (intact or cut cord) in babies ≥ 28 weeks gestation. Cord milking should be avoided in infant < 28 weeks gestation.
- Resuscitation with an intact cord if equipment, training, etc., allow for this.
- In some cases, ICC may be necessary.

My key take-home messages from this chapter are:

Airway management and ventilation

Introduction

Along with maintenance of temperature, management of the airway and support of breathing are the most important skills required in helping babies at birth.

This chapter discusses the following two key elements:

- how to open an airway, and once open
- how to inflate (aerate) the lungs and support breathing (if this is required).

Most babies do not need help with breathing at birth, but a small number do. The most commonly encountered situation is the hypoxic baby who has become unconscious and as a result has lost its respiratory drive and has floppy obstructed airways. Other scenarios (Table 7.1) are less common.

Table 7.1   Reasons for difficulties with breathing at birth

1. Loss of respiratory drive	
Acquired depression of the neurological centres responsible for initiating breathing in the unconscious baby	• Perinatal stress & hypoxia • Drugs e.g. maternal sedation/analgesia • Infection
Congenital brain abnormality	
2. Mechanical obstruction of the airway	
Loss of muscular tone affecting patency of the airway	• Unconscious baby (most common) • Congenital conditions affecting muscles
Foreign body	• Meconium, vernix, blood, mucus plug
Anatomical abnormality of the airway	• Pierre-Robin sequence and similar conditions
3. Inability to breathe	
Neurological and muscular conditions affecting the ability to breathe	
Lung immaturity	Preterm birth

The approach to managing the newborn airway, and the steps taken, is the same regardless of the cause.

Anatomical considerations

The airway of a newborn baby is different to the adult airway in ways which make it more vulnerable to mechanical obstruction. The tongue is proportionally larger, taking up more space in the mouth. The larynx is more anterior and the pharynx is tapered towards the cords like a funnel. In the unconscious baby with reduced tone, lying on their back, the pharynx tends to collapse, and both the jaw and tongue to fall back, obstructing the airway.

Matters are further compounded by the shape of the newborn head. The occiput is relatively large, especially after a normal delivery where cranial moulding exaggerates this tendency. The large occiput causes the neck to flex when the baby is placed supine on a flat surface, further compressing airway structures and obstructing the airway.

Opening the airway

The obstruction caused by the tendency of the pharynx to collapse and the tongue to fall back obstructing the airway in the unconscious baby lying on its back can be overcome by lifting the jaw (and thus the base of the tongue) forward.

Two manoeuvres can be used to ensure an open airway in an unconscious baby:

1. Hold the head in the neutral position with chin and jaw support.
2. Move the jaw forward using a two-handed jaw thrust.

Mask inflation will not work unless the airway is open.

Head position

To overcome the tendency of the neck to flex due to the prominence of the occiput when the floppy newborn baby is placed on its back (supine) you should place the baby's head in the neutral position with the neck neither extended nor flexed (Figure 7.1). If the baby is on a flat surface, then the neutral position can be easily achieved by placing a small (~2 cm thick) pad under the baby's shoulders.

The commonest reason for failure to open the airway is incorrect positioning of the neck, usually overextension.

Chin support and jaw thrust

In a baby with poor tone who is breathing, it will be necessary to support the chin using a finger on the bony part of the chin near the tip (Figure 7.2). Avoid pressing on the soft tissue under the chin as this may push the tongue base backwards and worsen the situation.

If the baby is very floppy, it may be necessary to use one or two fingers under each side of the lower jaw at its angle to push the jaw forwards (Figure 7.3). This is called a jaw thrust manoeuvre. It requires two hands, but it is the most effective method of opening the airway where two or more people are in attendance. If a mask is applied to the face, the jaw must always be supported by either chin support or jaw thrust.

In the conscious, or semi-conscious, baby who is trying to breathe, the manoeuvres described above may be sufficient to enable the baby's own breathing efforts to be effective. If the heart rate is adequate, no further intervention may be necessary. If the baby is not breathing, then the situation will not improve without additional intervention; then the baby needs help with lung inflation and breathing.

Figure 7.1	Hold the head in the neutral position

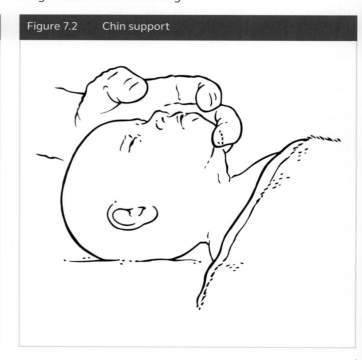

Figure 7.2	Chin support

Achieving transition to breathing via the lungs

Until the baby takes its first breath the lungs are filled with fluid. In fetal life, the lung secretes large quantities of fluid which pass out into the amniotic cavity.[84] In all mammals studied, the volume of fluid in the lungs at birth is about 30 mL kg^{-1}; this equates to ~100 mL in the average term baby.

At the onset of labour, various hormonal changes result in cells within the fetal lung switching from secreting to absorbing fluid.[180] A small amount of fluid, estimated to be 35 mL or so in a term baby, is expelled via the oropharynx during the passage through the birth canal. After delivery, the fluid in the alveolar spaces is pushed into the interstitial tissue of the lungs due to pressure generated by the baby taking its first breaths. The fluid is then absorbed into the lymphatic system over the next few hours to complete transition from intrauterine to extrauterine life (see Chapter 4 for more details).[98,99]

Babies who are born by caesarean section prior to the onset of labour will not have had the same physiological cues as those who experience the onset of labour, and this may go some way to explaining why such babies have a higher incidence of respiratory problems.[181]

Healthy, vigorous babies can achieve lung aeration with their first breath using negative pressures of around minus 30 cm water, but frequently less than minus 20 cm water.[182] Well babies can achieve a resting lung volume of 15–30 mL with the first breath. Once a breath has been taken, intrathoracic pressure is then often raised by crying to levels of 30–90 cm water. This probably helps to move lung fluid into the pulmonary interstitial tissues during the first few breaths.[66]

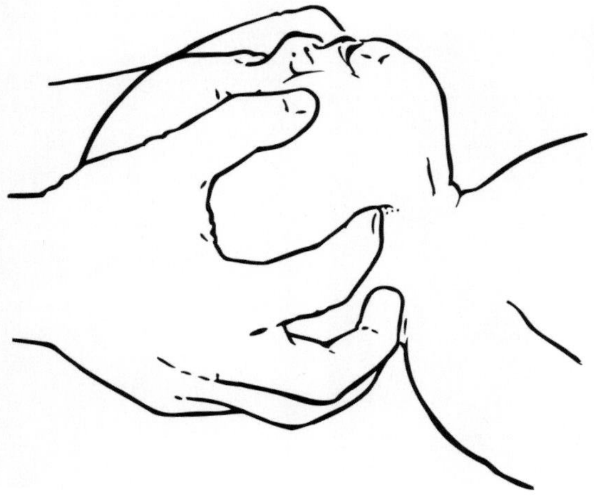

Babies needing resuscitation at birth, who have not breathed effectively for themselves, need help in achieving a resting lung volume. If positive pressure ventilation is used, then an inflation time of 2–3 s is required to inflate the lungs of a newborn baby.[138] When ventilating using positive pressure, gas will not enter the lung until it reaches a pressure above the 'opening pressure' of the lungs. Theoretical calculations from measurements in isolated lungs, as well as data from newborn babies, suggest that the opening pressure in babies needing resuscitation is 15–30 cm water (1.5–2.9 kPa) with a mean of about 20 cm water.[183]

In term babies needing resuscitation we recommend using an inflation pressure of 30 cm water, applied for 2–3 s (and repeated five times) to adequately inflate the lungs. For preterm babies we recommend these breaths are given using an initial lower pressure of 25 cm water.[31] Sustained breaths (of longer duration than 5 s) have not been shown to be of benefit[184] and one trial suggested they may cause harm.[185]

In some circumstances, a higher opening pressure may be required to overcome the opening pressure of particularly stiff lungs. If the appropriate airway-opening manoeuvres are being performed correctly, increasing the pressure applied in small, stepwise increments (2–5 cm water) may be beneficial. This should be supervised by a senior clinician and, importantly, once the opening resistance has been overcome, it is best practice to proactively reduce the pressures used in order to avoid barotrauma. Lung inflation is difficult to measure directly; but use of adjuncts such as a saturation monitor to give a continuous heart rate and oxygen saturation readings and end-tidal CO_2 monitoring will assist in judging if the airway opening manoeuvres and applied ventilation have been successful.

Equipment for positive pressure ventilation

Either a T-piece resuscitator device or self-inflating bag may be used to provide the flow of gas through the mask to the baby.

Never connect a device directly to a wall or cylinder-mounted flowmeter without a suitable blow-off valve in the circuit.

The self-inflating bag is often harder to use than the T-piece, and even with a PEEP (positive end expiratory) valve attached it will not deliver consistent PEEP.[186] Most self-inflating bags do not have a PEEP valve as part of the standard setup.

The T-piece device will deliver a more reliable PEEP and consistent peak inspiratory pressure. However, the T-piece is gas-driven and relies on a source of pressurised gas being available. In environments where there is no flow of high-pressure gas to allow the T-piece to work (such as in the community setting for a home birth), or where the gas flow fails (such as in an emergency on delivery

Figure 7.3   Jaw thrust

> **Figure 7.4** A T-piece system showing manometer and peak pressure blow off valve (far left), an air-oxygen blender (left) and T-piece with PEEP valve (right) attached to face mask

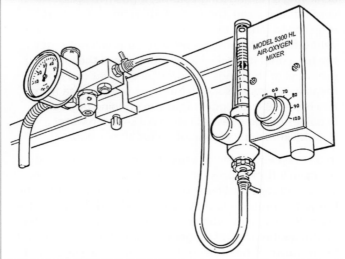
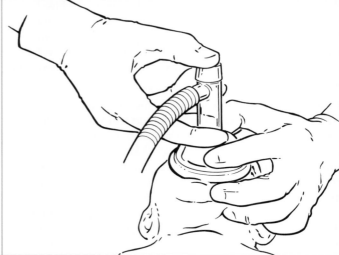

suite), the self-inflating bag provides a useful alternative to the T-piece. As the technique for using these devices is different, NLS providers should be familiar with the characteristics of both.[187,188]

The essential pre-requisites for **both** techniques are:

- an open airway
- a good seal between the mask and the baby's face.

T-piece

A soft, close-fitting face mask, a supply of pressurised gas, and an adjustable pressure release ('blow-off') valve (Figure 7.4) will allow positive pressure breaths to be administered to a baby. T-piece circuits also provide PEEP, usually via an adjustable valve on the T-piece turret. T-piece resuscitator circuits allow the peak inspiratory pressures to be adjusted by the operator as appropriate for the baby being supported and include an air-oxygen blender to allow titration of oxygen as required.

Self-inflating bags

These can be used to deliver inspiratory pressure in much the same way as a T-piece. They can be used where there is no piped or pressurised gas supply but delivering consistent positive pressure and PEEP is much more difficult. Self-inflating bags are discussed in more detail in Appendix 3.

Choosing and applying a mask

Using a face mask to allow inflation and ongoing ventilation of the lungs of a newborn is a skill that should be acquired by all involved in the care of the newborn. It can be difficult to do well however, and requires regular practice. It is easiest to obtain a seal with a silicone mask with a broad, soft deformable sealing surface or flange but anatomical masks with a cushion can work as well (Figure 7.5a).[189-192]

> **Figure 7.5a** Commonly used face masks for term babies from different manufacturers

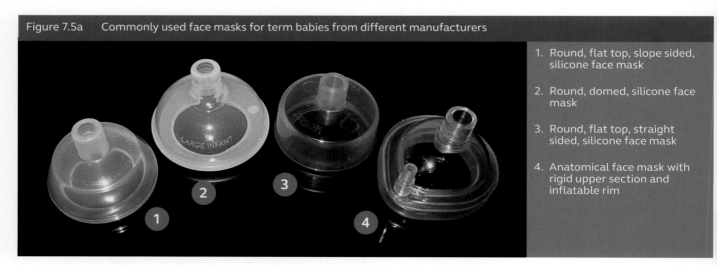

1. Round, flat top, slope sided, silicone face mask

2. Round, domed, silicone face mask

3. Round, flat top, straight sided, silicone face mask

4. Anatomical face mask with rigid upper section and inflatable rim

The soft deformable flange of a silicone mask is designed to mould around the baby's face to create an airtight seal during application of positive pressure. When such masks are applied to the face, force should be applied down through the mask with fingers holding the thickened upper section and avoiding the rim, which if squeezed may deform to break the seal against the face. Beware of applying excessive force, which may be uncomfortable for the baby and also deform the mask and create a less effective seal.

Other masks have a rigid upper section and a soft inflatable cushion. It is important to ensure the cushion is inflated, but not excessively so. Once again, the mask is held by the rigid upper section and it is the force applied through the mask which pushes the cushion against the face to make a seal.

The mask should cover the nose and mouth but should not extend over the edge of the chin and nor should it encroach on the orbits. Table 7.2 gives suggested mask sizes. Failure to achieve an airtight seal between the mask and the face is the commonest reason for failure of mask ventilation. Overestimating the size of the mask needed is a common reason for failing to achieve an adequate seal; sizing the mask properly to the baby's face is essential to prevent this, and it is often found that a smaller than anticipated mask will fit a given baby correctly during sizing. Unsurprisingly, small babies require small masks for ventilation (Figure 7.5b).

After correctly sizing the mask there are three key elements (the 3 Ps) to minimising face mask leak:

The 3 Ps

1 **Position:** rolling the mask onto the face ('align, roll, check') for a correct mask position (Figure 7.6a–b).

2 **Pressure**: balancing the pressure exerted on the mask by the finger and thumb (Figure 7.7).

3 **Pull:** lifting or pulling the jaw upwards into the mask (Figure 7.8).

These three steps used correctly can ensure that an effective mask seal is created; they can be applied to any mask design, term and preterm resuscitation and single resuscitator or two-person techniques.

Having done this:

- Further re-check the 3 Ps:
  - Position
  - Pressure
  - Pulling the jaw up.
- Re-check the airway position: is the head still in the neutral position?
- Then give inflation breaths.

Table 7.2 Estimating face mask size by gestation and/or birthweight (adapted from O'Shea et al[193] and Haase et al[194])

Gestation	Mask size	Weight g
23 weeks	35 mm	< 1000 g
24 weeks		
25 weeks		
26 weeks		
27 weeks	35 or 42 mm	1000–1249 g
28 weeks		
29 weeks	42 mm	1250–2000 g
30 weeks		
31 weeks		
32 weeks		
33–34 weeks	42 or 50 mm	2000–2499 g
35–36 weeks		
37 weeks	50 mm	< 3000 g
Term IUGR/38 weeks	50 or 60 mm	> 3000 g
> 39 weeks/LGA	60 mm	> 3500 g
Note: 50 mm = size 0/0 or size 0, and 60 mm = size 0/1 or size 1, dependent on manufacturer		

Figure 7.5b   Common preterm mask designs showing variation in sizes

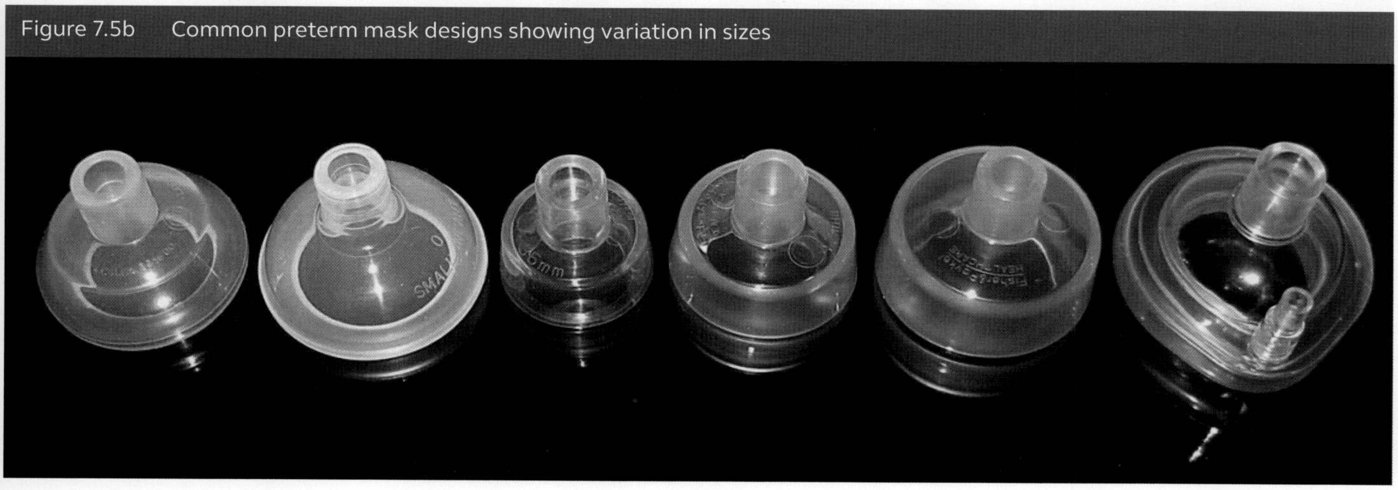

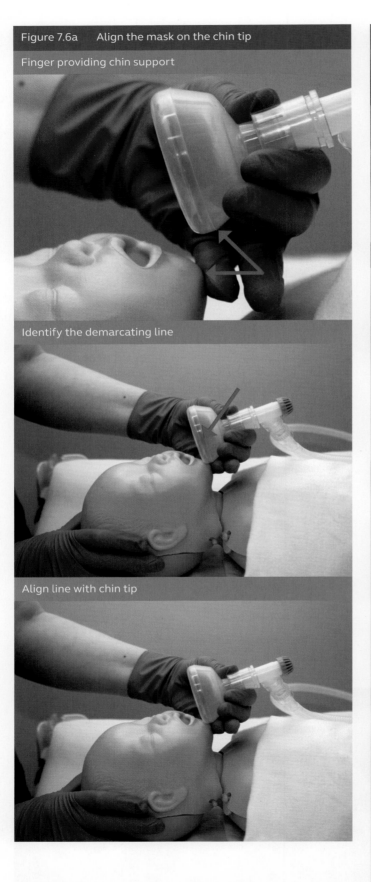

Figure 7.6a   Align the mask on the chin tip

Finger providing chin support

Identify the demarcating line

Align line with chin tip

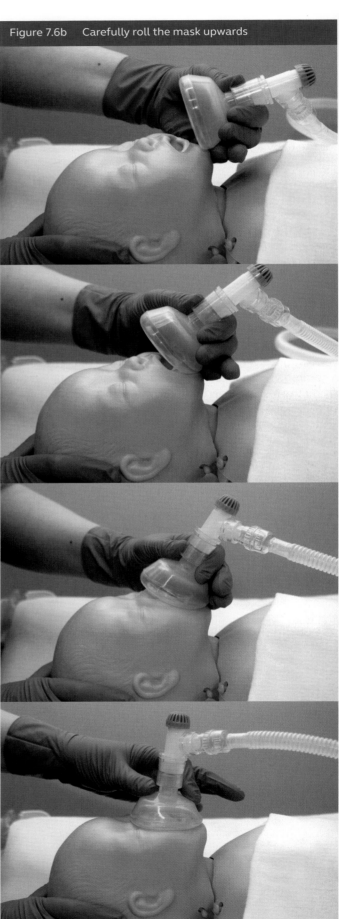

Figure 7.6b   Carefully roll the mask upwards

The 3 Ps

1 Position: rolling the mask onto the face ('align, roll, check') for a correct mask position (Figure 7.6a–b).

2 Pressure: balancing the pressure exerted on the mask by the finger and thumb (Figure 7.7).

3 Pull: lifting or pulling the jaw upwards into the mask (Figure 7.8).

Holding the face mask

There are a number of ways to hold the face mask (Figure 7.9); the key attribute of all these methods is that they ensure even pressure on the top of the mask without deforming the cuff of the silicone type masks.[195]

If the operator's hands are of sufficient size, then placing the thenar eminence (heel of the hand) on the left side of the forehead of the baby helps achieve stability.

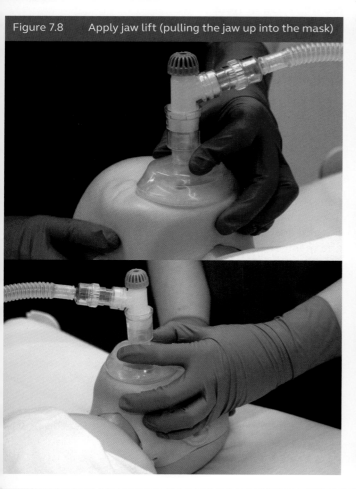

Figure 7.7   Carefully check the mask position and balance pressure exerted on the mask by the finger and thumb

Figure 7.8   Apply jaw lift (pulling the jaw up into the mask)

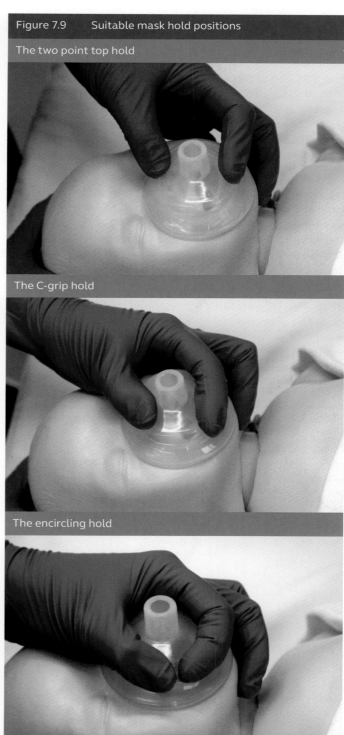

Figure 7.9   Suitable mask hold positions

The two point top hold

The C-grip hold

The encircling hold

Give inflation breaths

To inflate the lungs in a term baby, who is not breathing effectively for themselves, give five inflation breaths, maintaining the inflation pressure at about 30 cm water for 2–3 s with each breath. Too low a pressure is ineffective and too high a pressure can be dangerous. If there is a blender in the circuit it should usually be set to **AIR** in the first instance. Modifications for preterm babies are a lower initial inspiratory pressure of 25 cm water (< 32 weeks) and initial oxygen of 21–30% (28–32 weeks gestation) or 30% (< 28 weeks gestation). These starting parameters for oxygen and inspiratory pressure are summarised in Table 7.3.

The first two or three breaths will merely replace fluid with air without changing the volume of the chest. Therefore, you would not expect the chest to move until the fourth or fifth breath. After the first five successful inflations the lungs will be inflated and further ventilation can be managed with lower pressures.

Lung inflation is more easily achieved with a constant-flow pressure-limited device which can deliver Positive End Expiratory Pressure (PEEP), such as a T-piece system, than a self-inflating bag. Inflation breaths of 2–3 s to expand the lungs of the unconscious baby at birth are less easily achieved with self-inflating bag-mask systems.

A secure airway can be provided by insertion of a laryngeal mask device (see later in Chapter 7) or intubation (Appendix B) and may help to free NLS providers from the airway to concentrate on other issues if needed. However, these procedures must be carried out correctly with reliable fixation or they may adversely impact the ongoing ventilation of the lungs and be, in turn, less effective than good mask ventilation.

Table 7.3   Inflate the lungs with five 'inflation breaths' and begin with:

Gestation of baby	Starting oxygen concentration	Starting inflation pressure
Term	Air	30 cm water
32+0–36+6 weeks	Air	30 cm water
28+0–31+6 weeks	21–30% oxygen	25 cm water
Less than 28+0 weeks	30% oxygen	25 cm water

Check for a response

If you have successfully inflated the lungs and if the heart can respond then you will, in most cases, detect an increase in the baby's heart rate within 30 s. The heart rate response may, in preterm babies, be slightly slower. Therefore, if an increase in the heart rate is detected and maintained you can assume lung aeration has been successful.

> The first response to successful lung inflation and aeration is an increase in heart rate.

If the heart rate **does not** increase, this usually means that you have not successfully aerated the lungs. In some cases, however, it may mean that you have aerated the lungs but the heart cannot respond. If the heart rate does not respond to inflation breaths, the only way to check that the lungs have been aerated successfully is to see the chest move in response to your inflation breaths.

If the heart rate increases

If the heart rate has increased satisfactorily, then interventions have been successful, and no further inflation breaths are required. If the baby is not breathing, continued respiratory support with **ventilation** breaths are needed.

No increase in heart rate? – look for chest movement

If you **have** seen chest movement during your inflation breaths and the heart rate has not increased, deliver **ventilation** breaths at a rate of 30 min^{-1} and then reassess.

If you **have not** seen chest movement recheck the head position and face mask placement and repeat the **inflation** breaths, paying close attention to the chest movement.

When trying to deliver breaths to the lungs always be mindful of the position of the baby's head and jaw. Any baby hypoxic enough to require urgent resuscitation is likely to be unconscious and as limp as a patient under general anaesthesia, so the airway needs to be guarded and maintained. Use the airway opening manoeuvres described previously and recheck the position. If you do not have a second person to help, check the head is in the neutral position in case it has moved; ensure that adequate jaw thrust has been provided and repeat the five inflation breaths.

If you do not see chest movement after the second set of five inflation breaths, the most likely reason is that the airway is obstructed either because the head is not in the neutral position or because the jaw has not been drawn forwards. Two-person airway control or an airway adjunct such as a laryngeal mask can be very helpful at this point. Only rarely is the airway blocked by mucus, vernix, blood or meconium.

Figure 7.10   Different face mask holds that can be used when giving using a two-person jaw thrust

Four-point top-hold with jaw support

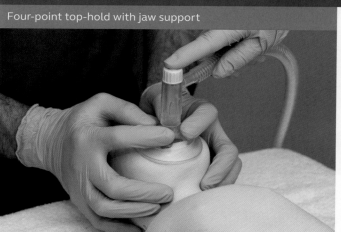

Two-thumb hold with jaw support

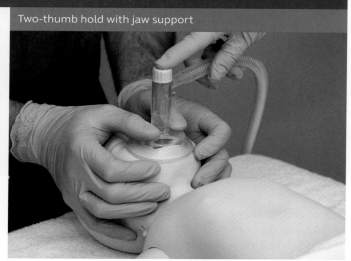

If there is no visible chest movement then there may have been no lung inflation.

Check the head position – reposition if needed – and repeat 5 inflation breaths.

Always check heart rate and chest movement after every manoeuvre.

Use two people (two-person airway support)

It is much easier to give mask inflation with two people.[197] One person stands (or kneels) at the baby's head, holding the head in the neutral position while applying a jaw thrust and concentrating on making a good seal with the mask. The two techniques for holding the face mask are shown in Figure 7.10. The second person occludes the T-piece or squeezes the bag.

Use of airway adjuncts

Airway adjuncts are devices to help the NLS provider manage the airway in a newborn baby and can be especially useful when only one provider is present where it is helpful to 'free up' a pair of hands (for example, to do cardiac compressions) or where there is an anatomically challenging airway.

Use of a laryngeal mask (supraglottic airway)

Laryngeal masks, also known as supraglottic airway devices, such as the laryngeal mask airway (LMA) or i-gel, have been used with good effect in babies whose weight is > 2000g or who are over a gestational age at birth of around 34 weeks. A variety of devices are available.[198] Anecdotal reports of use, with varying success, below these weights/gestations also exist.[199,200] There do not exist, at present, smaller laryngeal mask devices designed for use in very preterm babies.

Laryngeal masks work by providing a seal around the glottic opening, allowing a more direct application of ventilatory gas-flow into the trachea. Most laryngeal masks use an inflatable cuff to create a seal within the airway and prevent leak; the i-gel has a deformable mask shape which, when warmed by the surrounding tissue, gently moulds to the airway to create the seal.[198] Once in place, laryngeal masks can be fixed in a similar fashion to a tracheal tube to provide a more secure airway for a prolonged resuscitation. Laryngeal masks can effectively bypass abnormal face shapes or jaw sizes that might make mask ventilation difficult. Similarly they can be a helpful alternative to intubation when face shape or jaw size makes intubation harder. Consequently they are very useful in managing difficult airway. Laryngeal masks and other supraglottic airways (e.g. oropharyngeal and nasopharyngeal airways) appear to be well tolerated by babies.

When to use a laryngeal mask

Although laryngeal masks appear an attractive alternative, in the UK face masks remain the equipment of choice in the initial stages of respiratory support for babies, especially given the limitations of sizes available of laryngeal masks.

Laryngeal masks will, nonetheless, have a place in newborn resuscitation when:

- Face mask ventilation by skilled practitioners is found to be difficult.

- A degree of airway security is needed (e.g. during a prolonged resuscitation) and intubation is not possible (e.g. no-one available who is suitably trained or the intubation is technically difficult).

- The attendant is less experienced in providing mask ventilation to term and near-term babies (e.g. in a pre-hospital environment).

- To secure the airway whilst moving the baby e.g. transfer to NNU, transfer into hospital from home.

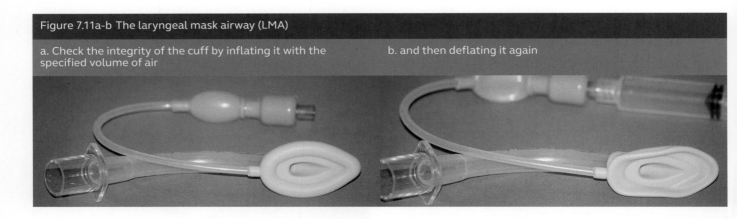

Figure 7.11a-b The laryngeal mask airway (LMA)

a. Check the integrity of the cuff by inflating it with the specified volume of air

b. and then deflating it again

Although face masks are the primary means of providing respiratory support in the UK, laryngeal masks have been shown in a low-resource setting to be an acceptable and equally effective alternative to face mask ventilation in the first-line support of babies requiring resuscitation.[201] Where respiratory support is infrequently given and the attendants less experienced, effective use can be taught more easily than mask ventilation.[202] The skills needed to successfully insert any laryngeal mask can be taught using a neonatal manikin; after viewing a 15 minute educational session using a manikin most people can insert a laryngeal mask in 15 s or less.[203]

Choosing and inserting a laryngeal mask

For babies, the correct size of laryngeal mask (in absence of smaller devices) will be a 'size 1' (for both LMAs and i-gels). Both devices are inserted in the same way with the mask opening facing upwards, and the device inserted in the same orientation in which it is to lie once in the baby's pharynx.

It is recommended that a laryngoscope is used to help to move the tongue and jaw to optimise mouth opening, and then the device is inserted sliding over the tongue until it meets resistance.

Once in this position, the LMA requires the cuff to be inflated (it will 'bounce' up a little), but the i-gel mask will soften with body heat and mould to the structures around the glottis. Once in place, the T-piece or self-inflating bag can be attached and breaths delivered. If the chest moves, the airway should be secured. If it does not, then the device should be checked for correct placement, and removal considered. In-line CO_2 detection may be used to assess whether there is some degree of effective lung ventilation with the laryngeal mask in place.

Inserting an LMA

- If the laryngeal mask has a cuff, check that it inflates and deflates correctly (Figure 7.11a & b).
- Lubricate the laryngeal mask with water soluble gel.
- The laryngeal mask is held so that the opening is in a forward-facing position (i.e. towards the baby's feet).
- The laryngeal mask is held 'like a pen' in the operator's dominant hand with the index finger placed just above the cuff. The device is inserted with the cuff deflated (Figure 7.11c).
- Position the head in a slightly extended position and use a laryngoscope to help move the tongue out of the way and create space for the laryngeal mask to pass.
- Introduce the laryngeal mask into the mouth. Slide the laryngeal mask downwards and backwards along the hard palate, to reach a resting position beyond the base of the tongue. A slight resistance to any further advancement will be felt (Figure 7.11d). A two-person jaw thrust may be applied during insertion to help if it is felt that the laryngeal mask is not passing easily.
- Once positioned, the cuff, if present, should be inflated using an air-filled syringe. A slight outward movement of the laryngeal mask will be observed when the cuff is inflated (Figure 7.11e).
- A manual ventilation device attached to the laryngeal mask should achieve chest movement in the normal manner (Figure 7.11f). An in-line CO_2 detection may be used to assess whether there is some degree of effective lung ventilation with the laryngeal mask in place.
- The laryngeal mask should be secured in place using soft tape or ties.
- If the laryngeal mask has not been successfully inserted after 30 s of trying, the baby should be ventilated using a face mask before re-attempting laryngeal mask insertion.

Figure 7.11c-f   Insertion of the laryngeal mask airway (LMA)

c. Inserting the LMA with the cuff deflated

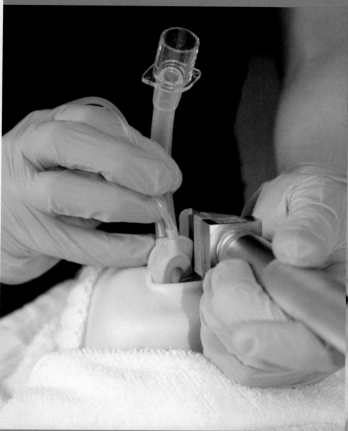

d. The LMA will meet with resistance once fully inserted

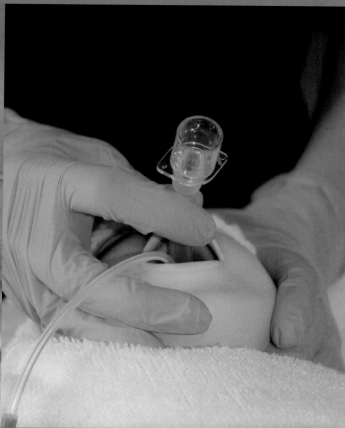

e. Reinflating the cuff of the LMA once in place

f. The T-piece being used with the LMA to ventilate the baby

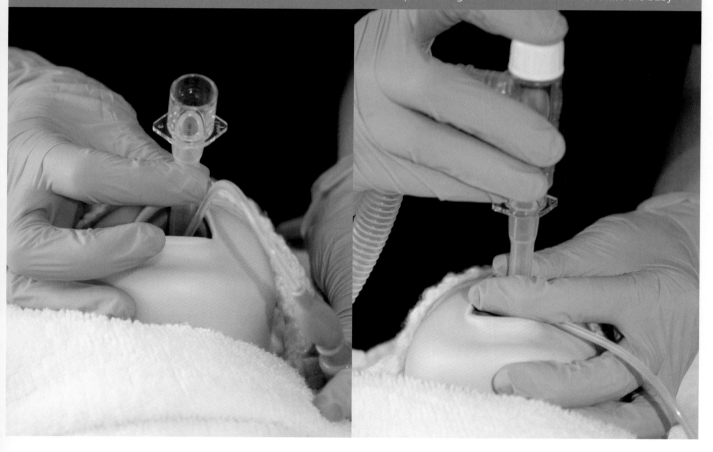

Figure 7.12a-b The i-gel

a. The standard laryngeal mask (top) and the i-gel. Both are supra-glottic airways; those pictured are both size 1 airways Both types have been used in babies larger than 2000 g

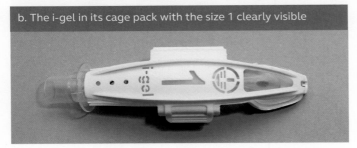

b. The i-gel in its cage pack with the size 1 clearly visible

Inserting the i-gel variant of laryngeal mask

The i-gel (Figures 7.12a-e) is a variation of the laryngeal mask that has a soft cuff that is not inflatable.[204] The soft cuff deforms to the shape of the airway at body temperature.

The i-gel comes in a cage pack with the size clearly marked (Figure 7.12b). The cuff of the i-gel should be lubricated with a small amount of water-based lubricant taking care to ensure that there is no bolus of lubricant left in the bowl of the cuff. The technique for insertion is similar to that described for the LMA except there is no balloon to inflate (Figures 7.12c–e).

The correctly inserted i-gel will protrude from the mouth slightly more than the corresponding similarly sized LMA due to the slightly longer overall dimensions (Figure 7.12e).

Figure 7.12c-e Insertion of the i-gel

c. Inserting an i-gel using a laryngoscope

d. Positioning the i-gel device

e. Using a T-piece to ventilate a baby via an i-gel

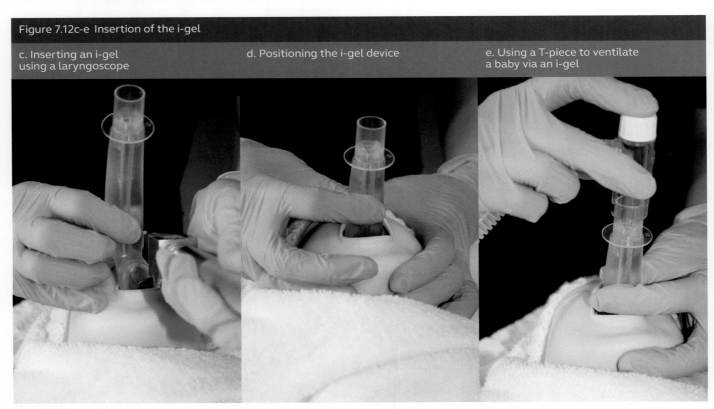

Use an oropharyngeal airway

An oropharyngeal airway (previously known as a Guedel airway) should always be available in settings where newborn babies may require assistance at birth. These are especially useful if there is some oro-facial abnormality affecting the airway. This can happen with a cleft palate – especially if there is micrognathia – or where the nasal passages are blocked or have not formed as in choanal atresia. Oropharyngeal airways can also be helpful when you are having difficulty providing both jaw thrust and mask inflation on your own and help is not immediately available. Under these circumstances an airway of the appropriate size will perform the same function as jaw thrust – that is support the tongue forwards out of the oropharynx.

> Note: Caution does need to be exercised with oropharyngeal airways as one RCT suggested that they may contribute to increased airway obstruction when used in preterm infants.[205]

Choosing an oropharyngeal airway

When using an oropharyngeal airway, it is important to choose the correct size. When held along the line of the lower jaw with the flange in the middle of the lips (immediately below the tip of the nose), the end of the airway should reach the angle of the jaw (Figure 7.13).

In babies and young children, the airway is inserted in the same orientation that it will finally lie. A laryngoscope (or tongue depressor if a laryngoscope is not available) should be used to hold the tongue out of the way during insertion (Figure 7.14). Make sure that the airway slips over the tongue and does not push the tongue backwards into the back of the mouth.

Sizing the oropharyngeal airway is only approximate and an assessment will also need to be made as the airway is inserted. Babies can vary in size from less than 500 to over 5000 g whereas there are only three sizes of neonatal oropharyngeal airway: 4, 5 and 6 cm. If the airway is too short, the distal end will impact on the base of the tongue and may be occluded. If the airway is too long, it may extend into the oropharynx below the tracheal opening and might obstruct the airway itself. The ideal length will reach just beyond the base of the tongue and will not protrude far out of the mouth in the unconscious baby.

Once inserted, reapply the face mask as previously described, re-establish the neutral position and give another five inflation breaths. Look for chest movement and check for an increase in heart rate. If the chest does not move or the oropharyngeal airway does not sit in the correct place when inserted, then the oropharyngeal airway should be removed before continuing.

If an airway is being considered, then it is both logical and pragmatic to have a look in the oropharynx at the same time as the laryngoscope is being used to control the tongue to exclude physical obstruction by particulate matter. A suction device should be ready to use in case particulate matter needs to be removed.

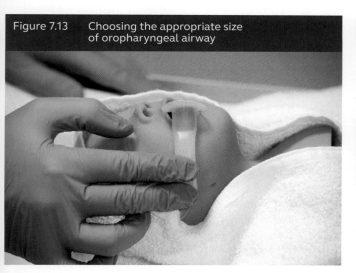

Figure 7.13 Choosing the appropriate size of oropharyngeal airway

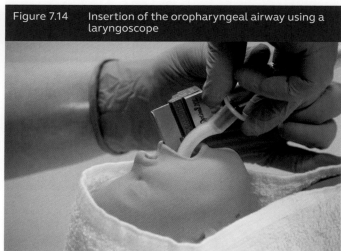

Figure 7.14 Insertion of the oropharyngeal airway using a laryngoscope

If the chest still won't move

When attempting lung inflation if the heart rate remains slow, and the chest does not move then the **AIRWAY** is the problem. When the more common causes (described above) have been ruled out consider airways obstruction even in the absence of meconium; inspect the airways and suction under direct vision. (See also Chapter 12 Babies who do not respond.)

Oropharyngeal obstruction

If the chest does not move with mask ventilation, especially after other airway manoeuvres, consideration should be given to there being an oropharyngeal blockage. The airway can be blocked by particulate matter such as meconium, vernix, blood or mucus. If inflation breaths do not work, consider using a laryngoscope to inspect the oropharynx and a large bore suction catheter to suction an obstruction.

Do not blindly insert a suction catheter into the mouth. Stimulation in the region of the posterior pharynx and larynx should be kept to a minimum because it easily induces adduction of the vocal cords and profound vagal bradycardia (though it will have little effect in a baby in terminal apnoea).

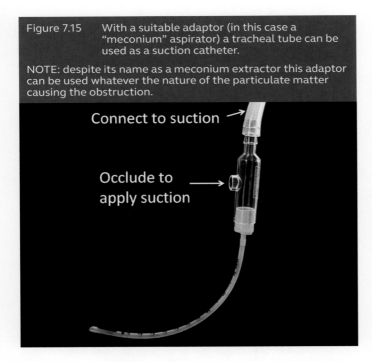

Figure 7.15   With a suitable adaptor (in this case a "meconium" aspirator) a tracheal tube can be used as a suction catheter.

NOTE: despite its name as a meconium extractor this adaptor can be used whatever the nature of the particulate matter causing the obstruction.

Connect to suction

Occlude to apply suction

Deep tracheal obstruction

Rarely, the trachea may be obstructed by such particulate matter aspirated before delivery or even after delivery. This can only be cleared by tracheal intubation and suction.

A baby gasping before or during delivery can inhale debris deep into the trachea. This can then block the trachea, frustrating attempts at lung inflation. If it is not possible to inflate the lungs despite airway opening manoeuvres, suction under direct vision and increased inflation pressures then senior help is needed urgently.

Material thick enough to cause airway obstruction cannot be sucked up any catheter small enough to be passed down inside a tracheal tube. A tracheal tube attached to a meconium aspirator should be used as a suction device (Figure 7.15). Otherwise, use the widest bore suction catheter available, preferably a 12 or 14 French gauge suction catheter, passed directly into the trachea.

Meconium-stained liquor

Lightly meconium-stained liquor is common and does not usually give rise to much difficulty during transition. The less common finding of very thick or particulate meconium-stained liquor at birth is an indicator of perinatal distress.

The normal intrauterine gentle 'breathing' efforts of a fetus are not sufficient to inhale particulate meconium in significant quantities. It is, therefore, reasonable to assume that if a baby has inhaled significant quantities of particulate meconium then that baby has been gasping. In other words, that baby has been stressed to such an extent that it has passed through primary apnoea and into the gasping phase before delivery. If that is the case, then the major determinants of the outcome for that baby are the circumstances and severity of the hypoxic insult that caused the baby to gasp rather than the meconium inhaled as a result of the gasping. This may be why several observational studies[135,206,207] and three small, randomised trials[208-210] of intubation and suction of the airways of **non-breathing** babies born through meconium-stained liquor have shown no benefit to this practice.

Most babies born through meconium-stained liquor have not inhaled any particulate material into the lower respiratory tract. If they have not done so as a result a period of anoxic gasping at birth they will only very rarely do so at birth. Large, multi-centre randomised studies have shown that the previously advocated practice of aspirating the airways of the emerging baby before delivery does not prevent the development of meconium aspiration syndrome[211] nor does routine tracheal suctioning of the airways of all babies (including those who are vigorous).[212]

There is increasing evidence suggesting that attempting to inspect the oropharynx or even intubate vigorous term babies is harmful. The most recent ILCOR Consensus on Science with Treatment Recommendations (CoSTR) recommends that initial resuscitative efforts are directed at inflating the lungs and that inspection of the oropharynx is considered only when lung inflation does not occur despite use of airway opening manoeuvres.[18] The emphasis, even when there is significant meconium-staining of the liquor, remains to open the airway, and quickly and effectively establish positive pressure respiratory support. This process should not be delayed for suctioning where meconium is present.

It is worth remembering that meconium is only one of several substances (others are blood, thick mucus, vernix) that may, on rare occasions, cause tracheal obstruction. If despite appropriate use of airway manoeuvres and adjuncts, the chest does not move and heart rate stays slow, prompt consideration should be given to one of these blocking the trachea.

The approach to a baby born through meconium-stained liquor

If a baby born through meconium-stained liquor is bradycardic and floppy, the emphasis is, in all cases, to inflate the lungs within the first minute after birth and this should not be delayed. Airway and tracheal obstruction due to meconium should be considered if the interventions described previously in this chapter have failed to generate a rise in either the baby's chest or heart rate. There is no evidence to support routine oropharyngeal or tracheal suctioning at birth in the absence of evidence that the airway is blocked – you cannot know this unless you have tried to inflate the chest.

In summary, the initial response to babies born through meconium-stained liquor should be:

Screaming babies	Have an open airway. You do not need to address any airway issues.
Floppy babies	Could potentially have a blocked airway however they should be treated according to the standard NLS algorithm. Dry and wrap. Then begin the standard airway opening manoeuvres and give inflation breaths. Consider airway suction if airway opening manoeuvres do not result in chest movement during inflation breaths.

Stiff lungs

The lungs of a sick newborn baby may sometimes be very stiff (i.e. the compliance is poor). There may have been suppression of endogenous surfactant production, or the lungs may have been afflicted with foreign matter such as meconium leading to decreased compliance.

In these cases, despite the manoeuvres discussed above it may not be possible to adequately inflate the lungs and oxygenate the baby. If the clinical situation suggests that stiff lungs may be a contributory factor, and you are confident that the airway is open, consider increasing the peak inflation pressure (in increments of 2–5 cm water). It would be very rare to need inspiratory pressures greater than 40 cm water, if increasing pressures senior help should be called.

This may be sufficient to exceed the higher critical opening pressure of the stiffer lung and enable lung inflation to occur. Once inflated, the pressures required to continue with ventilatory support may be lower. Be prepared to reduce the ventilation pressures as soon as possible. There is an increased risk of air leak or pneumothorax with such stiffer lungs, especially with higher pressures.

Oxygen and monitoring

Current evidence suggests that in babies > 32 weeks, resuscitation should start using air. In babies born between 28 and 32 weeks gestation, start resuscitation using an oxygen concentration between 21 and 30%. If the baby is less mature than 28 weeks, start with 30% oxygen.[31]

If resuscitation is prolonged, or there is a failure of the heart rate to respond to successful lung inflation, then consider increasing the inspired oxygen concentration. Use an oxygen saturation monitor early in such cases. Oxygen saturation monitoring also permits an estimation of the heart rate of the baby and, once stable, an indication of the level of oxygenation. Target right arm oxygen saturations are shown in Table 7.4. For babies < 32 weeks gestation, in particular, saturations of ≤ 80% at 5 minutes should be avoided.[213]

Outside labour ward most newborn resuscitations are performed using self-inflating bags. If oxygen is available, it is possible to increase the inspired oxygen to different levels (approximately 70% without using a reservoir bag[214,215] and nearly 100% if a reservoir bag is used[216]). If oxygen is not available continue ventilating with air.

Table 7.4 Target right arm oxygen saturations after birth

Time from birth	Acceptable (25th centile) right arm saturation
2 min	65%
5 min	85%
10 min	90%

Other approaches to opening the airway

The approaches described above will allow maintenance of the airway, inflation of the lungs and support of breathing in most situations. In prolonged resuscitations or other circumstances, a laryngeal mask or tracheal tube may allow the airway to be secured.

Other devices may also assist in establishing or securing an airway which allows either the baby to breathe effectively by themselves or face mask ventilation to work.

Nasopharyngeal airway (NPA)

Newborn babies are nasal breathers. If the nasal airway is compromised, they may struggle. The nasopharyngeal airway (NPA) works by splinting the airway from the nostril to the pharynx. It helps in situations where the upper airway is compromised because of functional obstruction of the nasal passages or posterior nasal space. A typical condition where this may arise is Pierre Robin sequence, where the small jaw and abnormally shaped tongue – coupled to a cleft palate leads to restriction of the posterior nasal space.

NPAs are simply flexible tubes which can be passed through the nostril and down past the tongue into the pharynx thus holding the airway open. Whilst there are specifically manufactured tubes for this purpose, a tracheal tube will suffice, ideally thin-walled to increase the effective internal diameter. The technique of choosing the correct size of and inserting the NPA is described in Appendix 2.

A note on tracheal intubation

There are few situations in which a baby must be intubated. However, intubation may be indicated for the further management of respiratory distress, upper airway abnormalities, prolonged apnoea, prolonged resuscitation, diaphragmatic hernia or to provide tracheal suctioning. The technique is beyond the Newborn Life Support course and, as a practical procedure, cannot be learnt from a manual, but the technique is described in Appendix B.

CPAP & PEEP from birth

Newborn babies who breathe spontaneously need to establish their functional residual capacity after birth. Failure to do this may lead to respiratory difficulties.[217] CPAP is the recommended method of respiratory support in spontaneously breathing preterm babies (Chapter 9) and may prevent the need for intubation and ventilation.[218]

Newborn babies of any gestation may show signs of respiratory distress such as grunting, nasal flaring, subcostal and intercostal indrawing, laboured breathing or persistent cyanosis. CPAP has increasingly been used to support more mature babies with such signs. However, there is little evidence to guide the use of CPAP in these more mature babies in the newborn period.[219,220] There are concerns from retrospective cohort studies that indiscriminate use of CPAP in near-term and term babies may lead to more pneumothoraces.[221-223]

Situations with minimal equipment

There are rare occasions when birth occurs in a setting where there is minimal or no equipment; in these situations, mouth-to-mask or mouth-to-mouth resuscitation can be used.

Mouth-to-mask resuscitation

If you happen to have an appropriately sized mask and no other equipment then mouth-to-mask resuscitation can also be effective. It allows you to apply two-handed jaw thrust while at the same time holding the mask in place before applying your mouth to the mask. The pocket mask is designed for use in this way with older children and adults.

Mouth-to-mouth resuscitation

Mouth-to-mouth (and nose) resuscitation is safe and it works. In larger babies mouth-to-nose resuscitation may be easier.[224] There remain the usual concerns regarding transmission of potentially serious infection either to or from the baby; use of appropriate equipment is always preferable. However, if equipment is not available it is certainly possible to resuscitate a baby at birth using this technique.

Having dried and covered the baby just remember to:

- Keep the upper airway open using head position and perhaps jaw thrust, as described earlier.
- Cover the baby's mouth and nose with your mouth (or close the baby's mouth and use the nose alone). Start with five inflation breaths of 2–3 s.
- Watch for chest movement and allow a little time for the lungs to empty before inflating the chest again. Once you have succeeded in inflating the chest, shorter breaths at a rate of 20–30 breaths min^{-1} are sufficient.

07: Summary learning

When attempting lung inflation...

- If the heart rate remains slow, and the chest does not move then the **airway** is the problem.

If the heart rate does not improve after five inflation breaths think:

- Is the baby's head in the neutral position?
- Do you need jaw thrust?
- Recheck the face mask position by repeating the align, roll and check process
- Are you using inflation breaths of 2–3 s?
- Do you need a second person's help with the airway?

Repeat the 5 inflation breaths. If the chest still does not move and heart rate slow:

- What about an airway adjunct (laryngeal mask, oropharyngeal airway)?
- Is there an obstruction in the oropharynx (laryngoscopy and suction)?
- Does the history suggest 'stiff lungs'?
  If so, consider increasing the inspiratory pressure in increments of 2–5 cm water.

If the chest still does not move:

- Consider deep tracheal obstruction even in the absence of meconium.
- Consider intubation if trained to do so.

My key take-home messages from this chapter are:

Circulation and drugs

Introduction

This chapter aims to provide an understanding of less frequently required aspects of resuscitation in the newborn infant; namely chest compressions and drugs. It covers some of the important practical aspects.

A **B** **C** **D**

Airway (A) and breathing (B) must be managed before circulation (C) and drugs (D). This chapter assumes that A & B have been managed and starts with chest compressions (circulation) and then follows with drugs. Without establishing an effective circulation, drugs will be ineffective.

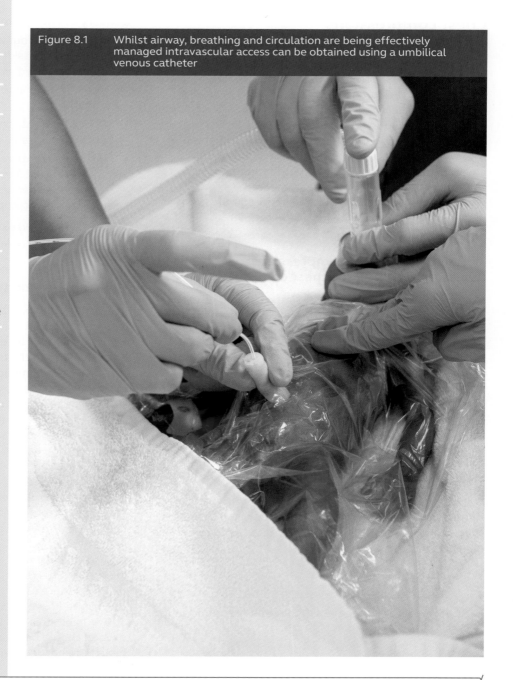

Figure 8.1   Whilst airway, breathing and circulation are being effectively managed intravascular access can be obtained using a umbilical venous catheter

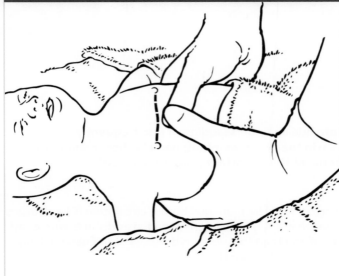

Figure 8.2   Two-thumb (two hand) chest compression

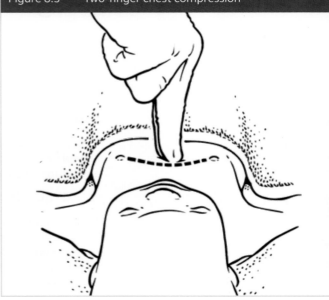

Figure 8.3   Two-finger chest compression

Chest compressions

If airway opening manoeuvres are successful and adequate lung inflation and ventilation is achieved, the need for chest compressions lessens. Observational studies suggest that approximately 85% term newborn babies begin breathing spontaneously; 10% will respond to drying, stimulation, opening the airway and/or applying CPAP or PEEP. Approximately 5% will breathe following positive pressure ventilation. Intubation, chest compressions or use of drugs are quite rare events; current intubation rates vary from 0.4% to 2%; fewer than 0.3% of babies receive chest compressions and approximately 0.05% (1 in 2000) receive adrenaline.[2,3,12,225,226]

When to start chest compressions: assessing the need for chest compressions

Circulatory support with chest compressions is effective only if the lungs have been successfully inflated and oxygen can be delivered to the heart. Ventilation may be compromised by compressions[227] and for this reason chest compressions are given in a synchronised way with ventilation breaths.[31]

It is rare for there to be no response to lung inflation at birth and the most likely reason for this is failure to aerate the lungs. You should address any issues with the airway as outlined in Chapter 7 before proceeding. When you have established an airway and seen chest rise during your inflation breaths, you should ensure that the chest is moving by ventilating for 30 s.

If the heart rate remains undetectable or very slow (less than 60 min⁻¹) after this, it is appropriate to provide chest compressions.[31]

When starting compressions

- Increase the inspired oxygen to 100%.
- Call for experienced help if not already summoned.

Delivery of chest compressions

- Synchronise your efforts so that you provide a cycle of three compressions to one ventilation breath at a rate of about 15 cycles every 30 s.
- Use a two-handed technique for compressions if possible.
- Check for a response every 30 s (or continuously if a pulse oximeter is available).
- If the heart rate remains very slow or absent, continue with a ratio of 3 compressions to one breath and secure the airway if not done already (e.g. consider intubation, if competent, or use of a laryngeal mask).

Titrate the inspired oxygen concentration against oxygen saturation once a reliable signal is achieved on the pulse oximeter.

What am I trying to achieve?

Resuscitating babies at birth is different from resuscitating adults. In adults you are usually dealing with a primary cardiac arrest and you need to keep oxygenated blood flowing to the brain and heart until the problem (e.g. arrhythmia, myocardial infarction) can be rectified. In the newborn baby, you have a healthy heart which has been pushed beyond normal physiological limits. You are merely trying to re-establish effective heart pumping, which should happen as soon as oxygenated blood reaches it; you can usually expect it to function virtually normally thereafter. This is important because even the best performed chest compressions can achieve only a fraction (approximately one third) of the cardiac output that is seen from a spontaneously and normally beating heart.[239,240] Preferential perfusion of the heart and brain in the hypoxic baby (Chapter 4) can improve the blood flow to these organs to approximately 50% of that seen in normal sinus rhythm provided effective resuscitation techniques are used.[241] If starting chest compressions, the inspired oxygen concentration should be increased to 100% unless this has already occurred. This supplemental oxygen should be weaned appropriately as soon as the heart rate has recovered.

Optimal method of chest compressions (two-thumb vs. two-finger technique)

Two methods[242] for performing chest compressions in newborn infants are commonly used; the two-thumb technique utilises the two thumbs to depress the sternum while the hands encircle the chest and the fingers may provide support behind the back (Figure 8.2) The two-finger technique utilises the tips of the middle and index fingers to depress the sternum and is easier in a single-person resuscitation scenario or if an umbilical venous catheter is being inserted (Figure 8.3).

Newer techniques, one using two thumbs at an angle of 90° to the chest and the other a 'knocking finger' technique, have been reported in manikins.[243] Further studies are required to determine if they have any clear advantage over the standard two-thumb technique.[18]

Existing studies suggest the two-thumb method is superior to the two-finger method; the two-thumb method with lateral chest wall compression (due to the encirclement of the chest) provided significantly higher mean, systolic, and diastolic blood pressures than the two-finger method.[244,245] Providers using the two-thumb technique were more likely to consistently provide compressions of the appropriate depth on manikins.[245] Delivering compressions using the two-thumb technique from 'over the head' appears as effective as the lateral position[246] and might be preferable to the two-finger technique when the umbilical venous catheter is being inserted.

Where should I press?

Compress the sternum over its lower third.[247,248] If you press too high on the sternum, the heart is not compressed; if you press too low, you risk damaging the liver. Place your thumbs or fingers on the sternum just below an imaginary line joining the nipples (Figures 8.1 and 8.2).

The two-thumb (two-handed) technique

Grip the chest in both hands, placing the thumbs together at the front with the fingers over the spine (Figure 8.1). Those with small hands may not be able to achieve this in larger infants and should position their thumbs as below first and then hold the side of the chest.

Your thumbs should be on the sternum and not on the ribs on either side. In performing the two-thumb technique, overlapping the thumbs on the sternum rather than placing them side-by-side provides better intrathoracic pressures for longer.[249] However, in a manikin study, overlapping the thumbs, whilst more effective than adjacent positioning, was found more likely to cause fatigue.[250] In a prolonged resuscitation this could be avoided by swapping out roles regularly.[251]

The two-finger technique

A less effective alternative method of chest compression[252] is to press at the same point on the sternum with two fingers (Figure 8.2). The back of the baby may need supporting if this manoeuvre is performed on a soft surface as this is less efficient (e.g. the baby can be pushed into the soft mattress).

This technique can be temporarily used to allow another person access to the umbilical cord in order to insert an umbilical venous catheter (UVC). Once the UVC is inserted, then ideally compressions should continue with the more effective two-thumb (two-handed) technique. A two-handed over-the-head technique has been described and assessed in manikin studies as a way of continuing this method during UVC insertion.[246]

How deep should I press?

It is recommended that chest compressions should be about a third of the depth of the chest. There continues to be an absence of specific data about ideal compression depth. It is important to realise it is a consensus opinion that one third of the depth of the chest would be appropriate and should be adequate to produce a palpable pulse.[252] Data from slightly older babies (median age one month) undergoing cardiac surgery suggests a depth of one half of the depth of the chest may be necessary,[253] but mathematical modelling based on chest CT scans supports that this may over-compress the heart in a significant proportion of babies.[254] What is clear from that is that a depth of less than one third is inadequate.

Chest compression in newborn babies does not cause rib fractures unless they have a rare severe bone disease such as osteogenesis imperfecta[255] and even then, it is not inevitable and should not deter from proceeding with chest compressions if they are needed.[149]

How do chest compressions work?

Although it was originally thought that the heart alone was emptied of blood during chest compression, it more likely that compression of the entire thorax is equally important. During the compression phase, blood is squeezed from the chest by the increased pressure in the thoracic cavity. The blood flows forward into the arteries rather than into the veins due to the venous valves at the thoracic inlet and because muscular walls keep the lumen of arteries patent whereas the thin-walled veins collapse.

It is important that there is enough time in the relaxation phase to allow the chest to refill with blood.[238] The cartilaginous rib cage of the newborn and the larger size of the heart relative to the chest make chest compression much easier as well as more efficient.

The history of chest compressions

In 1874, physiological studies first showed that directly squeezing the heart, in this case in a dog, could produce a cardiac output ('open chest cardiac massage').[228,229] Shortly afterwards, it was demonstrated that a similar effect could be produced by pressing on the sternum and the ribs without having to open the chest ('closed chest cardiac massage'[230]), and the successful use of such a technique in a human is attributed to Friedrich Maass in 1892.[231] Unfortunately, this technique was then forgotten for over 70 years before being 'accidentally rediscovered' during physiological investigations into the effects of defibrillation when Guy Knickerbocker noticed by chance that when he pressed electrode paddles firmly on the chest he could produce a rise in arterial pressure. This led to the rediscovery and reintroduction of chest compression to adult patient care as described in 1960 by William Kouwenhoven.[71]

At about the same time, interest was also being shown in the use of cardiac compressions during newborn resuscitation[232] and a number of reports of both 'open'[233] and 'closed'[72, 234-237] cardiac massage were published in the early 1960s. Not long afterwards, 'closed' massage, today known as chest compression, was being widely adopted.[236] The authors of early reports of closed chest compressions would probably recognise the techniques used today, albeit with some minor changes.

Because chest compressions are an infrequent event in newborn resuscitation there is very little scientific evidence behind the current recommendations for chest compressions in this situation. Most of the recommendations are extrapolations from animal, paediatric, and adult literature, as well as simple physiological plausibility and some expert opinion.

How fast should I press?

Current guidelines recommend synchronised chest compressions and ventilations in a ratio of 3:1 to achieve 90 compressions and 30 breaths (i.e. 120 events) in one minute.[18,31] This ratio is a consensus opinion, based on physiological plausibility and evidence supporting its use.

Both the compression and the recoil are important. You are not trying to reproduce a normal neonatal heart rate of about 140 min^{-1}. If you try to do so you will not produce effective blood flow because the technique is not as mechanically efficient as normal cardiac function. The rate you achieve is influenced by the chest wall compliance of the baby. Allow time after each compression for the chest to refill, by allowing it to re-expand fully. A compression to relaxation ratio with a slightly longer relaxation than compression phase offers theoretical advantages for blood flow in the very young.[256]

A 3:1 compression to ventilation ratio is used for resuscitation at birth where compromise of gas exchange is nearly always the primary cause of cardiovascular collapse. In one manikin study, a greater depth of compression was achieved, and operators were more likely to sustain the correct depth for longer, when using a 3:1 versus 15:2 ratio.[257] Minute ventilation is also greater.[258] A recent review of the evidence found no advantage of other ratios over the synchronised 3:1 technique in terms of time to the return of spontaneous circulation or other post-resuscitation parameters.[18,259] In practice, delivering chest compressions at this rate can be difficult to sustain.[260] In prolonged resuscitations, consider switching personnel before they fatigue to prevent deterioration in quality of compressions delivered.[251]

Rescuers may consider using higher ratios (e.g. 15:2) if the arrest is believed to be of cardiac origin, or in a postnatal collapse outside the maternity setting (e.g. the Emergency Department where staff may be more familiar with a 15:2 ratio).[31]

In the baby who has reached the stage of cardiac standstill, performing chest compressions without addressing the airway and breathing will simply result in the circulation of deoxygenated blood.[261,262] Establishing and maintaining effective ventilation is essential to any success.

When chest compressions are indicated by a persistent very slow/absent heart rate, guidelines recommend increasing the supplementary inspired oxygen to 100%.[31] in order to try and improve the oxygenation of the myocardium. However, there is no evidence to support this.[263-265]

If the baby has a laryngeal mask or tracheal tube placed, compressions and ventilations are continued using the same synchronised 3:1 ratio. Continuous, asynchronous chest compressions used in adults when intubated are not recommended in newborns. In a porcine model of newborn hypoxia, the potential for asynchronous compressions to interfere with ventilation was reflected in almost a third of breaths being affected by compressions, furthermore blood gas parameters after return of spontaneous circulation were worse.[266] Little is known about how asynchronous compressions would impact on breaths in the non-intubated baby receiving mask ventilation.

How long should I continue?

If it is going to, the heart rate should respond quickly to effective chest compressions, usually within 20–30 s.[12] Recheck the heart rate every 30 s to detect any response. If there is no response move on to administration of drugs and consider reasons for lack of a response (see below). If the heart rate is > 60 min⁻¹ and continuing to improve chest compressions can be stopped. However, regular reassessment must check that the heart rates continues to improve and chest compressions should be restarted if it drops below 60 min⁻¹.

What if I get no response?

The most likely reason for a lack of response to chest compressions is that the lungs have not been effectively aerated. Before using drugs check that the chest is definitely moving in response to ventilations delivered either by face mask, laryngeal mask or tracheal tube. Check that you are giving effective chest compressions. Drugs will not work if these are not being performed adequately.

When are drugs needed?

If you get no response to adequate chest compression combined with effective lung inflation and ventilation, resuscitation drugs should be used. The most likely reasons for the lack of response to inflation, ventilation and chest compressions are myocardial dysfunction secondary to lactic acidosis, pulseless electrical activity (formerly known as 'electro-mechanical dissociation') or possibly exhaustion of myocardial glycogen.

This is a rare event, occurring in approximately 0.05% (1 in 2000) of deliveries.[2,13,226] Although drugs have been used in this situation for decades there is very little human evidence that they are effective and, though some babies appear to respond initially, the outlook is generally very poor.[267] Some studies report better results but careful reading suggests drugs were sometimes used before effective airway management, inferring that these drugs were given unnecessarily.[268]

If you reach the point of requiring drugs consider other factors which may impact on the response to resuscitation such as equipment failure, pneumothorax, hypovolaemia and congenital abnormalities; these may need to be addressed before you see a response.

Routes of administration of drugs

Steps should be taken to secure vascular access. The umbilical vein offers rapid central vascular access in newborn babies and should be considered the primary method during resuscitation. Intraosseous (IO) access can be an alternative method of emergency access for drugs and fluids.[269,270] The intraosseous route may be useful in the very rare situation when a baby who has an abnormal umbilical cord and who also needs drugs during resuscitation.[271] In the absence of any vascular access, adrenaline may be given via a tracheal tube.[272,273] Drugs are unlikely to reach the heart after peripheral venous administration when there is complete circulatory arrest, even with good quality basic life support that includes chest compressions.

The history of umbilical vein catheterisation

Catheterisation of the umbilical vein to provide venous access for an exchange transfusion in cases of Rhesus disease was first reported in 1946.[274] Since then, umbilical vein catheters have been used to provide central access in sick babies for a variety of reasons including administration of inotropes, parenteral nutrition,[275] hypertonic solutions, angiography,[276] and blood sampling. The first published report of use during resuscitation did not appear until 1980.[277]

Drugs used during resuscitation

Drugs are rarely required during newborn resuscitation and the evidence for the efficacy of any drug is limited. The following drugs may be considered during resuscitation where, despite adequate control of the airway, effective ventilation and chest compressions for 30 s there is an inadequate response and the HR remains very slow or absent.[278] Adrenaline should be the first resuscitation drug given and should be repeated every 3–5 minutes if CPR is ongoing. Glucose is likely to be needed. Bicarbonate may be needed in a prolonged resuscitation (see Table 8.1, pragmatic drug doses may also be found in Table 8.2).

Adrenaline (epinephrine)

- when effective ventilation and chest compressions have failed to increase the heart rate above 60 min⁻¹

- intravenous is the preferred route, IO is an alternative:
  - give 20 micrograms kg⁻¹ (0.2 mL kg⁻¹ of 1:10 000 adrenaline (1000 micrograms in 10 mL))
  - a dose range 10–30 micrograms kg⁻¹ is acceptable which facilitates dosing based on estimated weight

- intra-tracheally if intubated and no other access available
  - at a dose of 100 micrograms kg⁻¹

- if intra-tracheal adrenaline is used and is ineffective then IV/IO access should be sought

- subsequent doses every 3–5 minutes if heart rate remains < 60 min⁻¹.

The history of adrenaline in resuscitation and evidence for its use

In the management of cardiac arrest, adrenaline acts via almost entirely via alpha-adrenergic receptor-mediated vasoconstriction[278] to elevate the aortic to right atrial pressure gradient during the relaxation phase of cardiopulmonary resuscitation.[279] This increases coronary artery perfusion pressure which, in cardiac arrest due to abnormal rhythms, is directly related to both myocardial blood flow and return of spontaneous circulation.[280]

The evidence for the most appropriate dose of adrenaline in any age group is sadly lacking; initial animal studies of adrenaline used an arbitrary dose of 1 mg (which approximated to about 0.1 mL kg⁻¹ in the dogs used in the studies).[279,281] A standard 1 mg dose was then adopted in adult humans which approximated a weight-based dose of 10 microgram kg⁻¹. This dose was subsequently adopted in paediatric and neonatal protocols despite the lack of any evidence.

Adult and paediatric protocols then started to recommend increasing the dose of adrenaline ten-fold (100 micrograms kg⁻¹) if there was no response to the initial 10 microgram kg⁻¹ dose, when evidence from animal studies suggested that higher doses led to improved cerebral and cardiac blood flow,[282] as well as improved return of spontaneous circulation.[283] The high doses were not adopted in newborn resuscitation for a variety of reasons; a multi-centre, randomised, double-blind trial of high (100 microgram kg⁻¹) versus standard dose (10 microgram kg⁻¹) adrenaline in children found a lower 24-hour survival for the high-dose group especially in those children whose arrest was secondary to hypoxia.[284] High dose adrenaline in neonatal piglets subjected to acute severe hypoxia showed no advantage in terms of survival at 24-hours, but caused tachycardia and systemic hypertension,[285] the latter is known to increase the risk of intraventricular haemorrhage.[286]

Animal evidence suggests adrenaline cannot bind to its receptors at very low pH.[287] If there is no response to a dose of 20 microgram kg⁻¹ it may be worth giving a dose of bicarbonate.

Unlike the other drugs mentioned in this section, adrenaline can be safely given down a tracheal tube.[288] However, the standard intravenous dose if given by this route is less effective due to the fetal lung fluid.[289,290] A higher dose of 100 microgram kg⁻¹ is recommended but the safety and efficacy of such a dose has not been determined. Use of standard doses via the umbilical venous or intraosseous route is preferred.

Glucose

- in a prolonged resuscitation to reduce likelihood of hypoglycaemia

- intravenous or intraosseous:
  - 250 mg kg⁻¹ bolus (2.5 mL kg⁻¹ of 10% glucose solution).

Glucose and evidence for its use

The heart cannot work without glucose and the glycogen stores present in the heart at birth are rapidly depleted during prolonged hypoxia. Babies being resuscitated will, prior to administration of glucose, have significantly lower blood glucose.[291] Glucose can be tried if there is no response to adrenaline. It is preferrable to use 10% glucose and subsequent symptomatic hypoglycaemia, if present, is better managed with an infusion of 10% glucose rather than with repeated boluses. **Glucose must never be given down the tracheal tube.**

During hypoxia, anaerobic metabolism and glycolysis rapidly depletes hepatic glycogen and glucose production rapidly becomes insufficient to meet cerebral metabolic demand. The evidence for the use of glucose in this situation is poor; however studies have shown a significant positive linear correlation between plasma glucose level and Apgar scores, and a significant negative linear correlation between the glucose level and severity of stages of hypoxic ischemic encephalopathy (HIE).[291]

A blood glucose level < 2.6 mmol L⁻¹ was reported in 25% of babies in the UK TOBY cooling registry,[292] and both hypoglycaemia and hyperglycaemia were associated with poorer neurological outcomes.[293] In babies with HIE, an abnormal early postnatal glycaemic profile (i.e. hypoglycaemia, hyperglycaemia or labile blood glucose) is associated with distinct patterns of brain injury on MRI.[294]

Administration of glucose is therefore logical in prolonged resuscitation and has been recommended in unresponsive newborn bradycardia or asystole. A glucose infusion should be considered in the post-resuscitation period.[18,31]

Table 8.2   Pragmatic resuscitation drug doses for a term baby

	Adrenaline (1 in 10,000)	Glucose (10% solution)	Volume (0.9% sodium chloride or blood)	Sodium bicarbonate (4.2% solution)
Suggested doses for a term baby*	0.7 mL	10 mL	35 mL	10 mL
Birth weight will not be known at the onset of newborn resuscitation and an estimated weight has to be used.				

Table 8.1   Neonatal resuscitation drug doses

Drug	Dose	Route	Comments
Adrenaline	0.2 mL kg^{-1} 1:10 000 (20 microgram kg^{-1})	IV/IO	Flush in adrenaline dose Repeat every 3-5 minutes
	1 mL kg^{-1} 1:10 000 (100 microgram kg^{-1})	Tracheal tube	Continue to seek vascular access
Glucose	2.5 mL kg^{-1} bolus 10% glucose (250 mg kg^{-1})	IV/IO	Useful in prolonged resuscitation Never give via tracheal tube
Volume	10 mL kg^{-1} 0.9% sodium chloride or O -ve blood	IV/IO	Slow bolus over ~2 minutes If suspected blood loss or unresponsive to other resuscitation measures
Sodium bicarbonate	1–2 mmol kg^{-1} sodium bicarbonate (2–4 mL kg^{-1} of 4.2% solution)	IV/IO	Slow IV injection 8.4% solution can be diluted with an equal volume of glucose to give 4.2% solution
All IV/IO drugs should be flushed with at least 2 mL of 0.9% sodium chloride IV: intravascular, the preferred vascular access route is a UVC IO: intraosseous, this is a secondary option			

Sodium bicarbonate

- may be considered in a prolonged unresponsive resuscitation with adequate ventilation, to reverse intracardiac acidosis
- intravenous or intraosseous:
  - 1–2 mmol kg^{-1} sodium bicarbonate (2–4 mL kg^{-1} of 4.2% solution) by slow intravenous injection.

NOTE: The widely available 8.4% sodium bicarbonate solution contains 1 mmol mL^{-1} and may be diluted with an equal volume of glucose to give a 4.2% solution.

Sodium bicarbonate and evidence for its use

There are several concerns about the use of sodium bicarbonate in babies[297] and its **routine** use during **brief** resuscitation is not recommended.

If there is no effective cardiac output, or virtually none, then reversing intracardiac acidosis may be helpful. This is certainly true in animal experiments.[52] You are not attempting to correct the baby's metabolic acidosis; you are merely trying to improve cardiac function by improving the pH of the blood within the heart.

An alkalising agent will normally produce cardiac acceleration within a couple of minutes if it is going to work. **Bicarbonate must never be given down the tracheal tube.**

Volume replacement

- with suspected blood loss or shock unresponsive to other resuscitative measures
- intravenous or intraosseous:
  - 10 mL kg^{-1} of group O Rh(D) negative blood or 0.9% sodium chloride
  - Give as a slow bolus over about 2 minutes.

Volume replacement and caveats

In the absence of blood loss, there is little evidence to support volume administration in the newborn baby with no blood loss who does not respond to ventilation, chest compressions and adrenaline. However, because blood loss may be occult, a trial of volume administration may be considered.

A bolus of about 10 mL kg^{-1} is usually sufficient to produce a response and can be repeated if necessary. If blood loss is the cause of the problem, further transfusion with blood may be necessary later. Giving further volume to a severely compromised baby with a myocardium damaged by hypoxia is likely to do more harm than good. Extreme caution should be exercised when giving volume to very preterm babies.[295] Giving large volumes (more than 40 mL kg^{-1}) of solutions high in chloride (such as albumin or 0.9% sodium chloride) can also exacerbate metabolic acidosis through hyperchloraemia.[296]

08: Summary learning

Use chest compressions when there is a very slow (< 60 min^{-1}) or undetectable heartbeat, but only after you have inflated the lungs and given 30 s of ventilation breaths.

Press down quickly and firmly, aiming to reduce the depth of the chest by about one third with each compression, and then release. Pause after each release to allow the chest to recoil fully.

Too rapid a compression rate gives the chambers of the heart no chance to refill passively after compression.

Synchronise 3 compressions with each ventilation (i.e. use a 3:1 ratio)

If the heart rate remains a very slow or undetectable despite 30 s of chest compression and adequate ventilation, consider drugs. Continue with ventilation and chest compressions.

An umbilical venous catheter (UVC) is the preferred way to give resuscitation drugs; intraosseous (IO) access is an alternative. Adrenaline is the only neonatal resuscitation drug that can be given via a tracheal tube but this route is not very effective.

If lung inflation and ventilation breaths followed by chest compressions are not working, then the outcome even with drugs is likely to be poor.

My key take-home messages from this chapter are:

Preterm babies

In this chapter

The learning outcomes will enable you to:

Appreciate that most preterm babies require help with transition rather than resuscitation

Understand how to support the transition of preterm babies

Understand why attention to thermal care is vital in these babies

Appreciate the importance of avoiding harm caused by hypothermia, hyperoxia, hyperventilation by using pulse oximetry to guide oxygen use

Understand the use of CPAP or, if required, gentle ventilation (lower inflation pressures, PEEP and prophylactic surfactant)

Degrees of maturity

Current accepted obstetric practice classifies babies as having reached 'term' (implying gestational maturity) when born between 37+0 weeks and 41+6 weeks, though the lowest risk of stillbirth occurs at 38 weeks.[298]

Most moderate and late preterm babies, term and post-term babies are unlikely to need significant assistance at delivery. The approach to stabilisation, if needed, follows the standard NLS algorithm. However, before 32+0 weeks gestation it is a different matter (Figure 9.1) and every effort should be made to ensure that an appropriately trained person is present at their delivery (see Chapter 6).

Table 9.1	Definitions of preterm birth
Extremely preterm	Born at less than 28+0 weeks gestation
Very preterm	Born between 28+0 and 31+6 weeks gestation
Moderately preterm	Born between 32+0 and 33+6 weeks gestation
Late preterm	Born between 34+0 and 36+6 weeks gestation
Post-term babies	Born at or after 42+0 weeks gestation

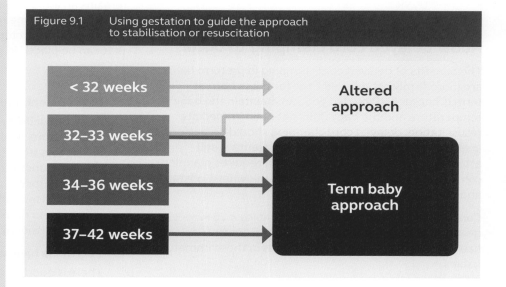

Figure 9.1   Using gestation to guide the approach to stabilisation or resuscitation

< 32 weeks → Altered approach

32–33 weeks

34–36 weeks → Term baby approach

37–42 weeks

Optimising place of delivery

A regional approach is required to ensure that the most vulnerable babies, for example, those who are born before 27 weeks, are offered the best perinatal care by transferring, antenatally if possible, to a specialist centre. The British Association of Perinatal Medicine have produced a framework for the perinatal management of babies < 27 weeks gestation.[144] This outlines an approach to counselling parents and weighing up the impact of starting intensive care, especially at extremely early gestations (22–23 weeks). These families need careful counselling by senior clinicians about whether to offer 'survival focused care' or 'comfort focused care' (Chapter 12).

Assisting transition rather than resuscitation

Most preterm babies are in reasonable condition at birth and are only in need of assisted transition, not resuscitation.[5] In other words, they are fragile individuals needing careful handling and gentle support, not critically ill babies on the point of death. Provided babies can be kept warm it is to their advantage that clamping of the cord is delayed and they remain attached to the placenta for a period while establishing pulmonary respiration.[170]

Allow delayed cord clamping to occur

The benefits of delayed cord clamping in preterm babies are more firmly established than for those born at term (Chapter 6). Provided you can maintain the baby's temperature and the baby does not need immediate resuscitation, delayed cord clamping should be performed in all preterm deliveries where the placenta is still attached to the uterus. This approach requires planning, communication and teamwork by all midwifery, obstetric and paediatric staff involved.

Cord milking should not be done in babies < 28+0 weeks gestation due to the increased risks of intraventricular haemorrhage that cord milking brings in these immature babies.

Keeping the baby warm – polythene bags and radiant heat

Why?

The preterm baby is particularly vulnerable to heat loss and subsequent hypothermia as they have immature thin skin, reduced subcutaneous fat, poor vasomotor control and an increased body surface to mass ratio.

There is an increased mortality associated with hypothermia, especially in small and preterm babies, and for every 1°C below 36.5°C the baseline risk of mortality increases by up to 28%.[32] Mortality is highest at lower admission temperatures, and admission temperatures less than 32.9°C have been associated with more than 80% mortality.[299] Even a brief period of hypothermia is associated with neonatal morbidity, impaired surfactant synthesis, impaired surfactant spreading within the lungs, pulmonary hypertension, hypoxia and coagulation defects. Acidosis and hypoxia further inhibit surfactant production.[27,300]

Hypothermia may be a marker for increased risk of death, especially in babies who continue to lose heat during stabilisation. Meticulous attention to temperature remains an integral part of the approach to the newborn preterm baby. Some resuscitation platforms allow servo-controlled temperature management with probes that can be placed in a number of locations.[301]

How?

1. **Environmental temperature**

   Raise the delivery room or operating theatre temperature, ideally to at least 26°C when managing babies less than 28 weeks gestation.[35,36] Achieving this in practice is not easy.[302] The piped gases used for respiratory support in the delivery room are cold and dry gases and can also contribute to heat loss. Heating and humidifying these gases improves the NNU admission temperatures in preterm babies.[303]

2. **Polythene bags under radiant heat**

   There is good evidence that it is easier to maintain the temperature of very preterm babies if they are placed immediately after birth, without drying, into a polythene bag.[304] It is important to remember that the babies in these studies were also then placed under a radiant heater.

   Some specially designed bags are available but any food grade bags may also be used; the face should not be covered but it is helpful to cover the baby's head with a hat. If you need access to areas of the baby within the polythene bag, a small cut can be made in the bag for this purpose. Once the baby is on the resuscitaire do not cover the polythene bag with anything else but leave directly under the radiant heater.

3. Polythene bags without radiant heat

The main advantage of using a polythene bag is that it substantially reduces evaporation from the surface of the baby. Wrapping a baby in polythene and then placing the baby next to a warm object, such as their mother's skin, and covering both with a warm towel will probably keep the baby warmer than a similar baby not covered in polythene, but the data is not available to prove this. This strategy could be employed for preterm babies delivered outside hospital as a means to keep them warm on the way to hospital.[305,306]

Early monitoring of the baby's temperature is recommended. Chemical thermal mattresses can be used to help maintain a preterm baby's temperature but care should be taken when using a chemical mattress in conjunction with a radiant heater, as overheating could occur.

Helping to establish pulmonary gas exchange

The lungs are fragile

The lungs of preterm babies are more fragile and less compliant than those of term babies, whilst at the same time their chest wall is more compliant and less able to protect the lung against over-inflation. Over-enthusiastic inflation of fragile lungs can predispose to serious inflammatory damage and long-term morbidity.[307] Assessing delivered tidal volumes without respiratory function monitors is very difficult.[308]

Most preterm babies are breathing after birth

Unlike the term baby who needs support at birth due to absence of any breathing, the majority of preterm babies will either cry, or at the very least breathe spontaneously without intervention.[309] They also have immature lungs and respiratory control mechanisms; therefore, they require support to ensure that effective breathing continues rather than actually requiring resuscitation. Non-invasive respiratory support, rather than intubation and ventilation, is the preferred method of supporting these babies.[310]

Whilst non-invasive respiratory support is generally effective, it requires skill and may be complicated by the leakage of gas around the mask making it less effective.[308] Using smaller face masks may not totally abolish the leak.[311] In addition, applying an interface such as a face mask may invoke immature reflexes in preterm babies that temporarily cause apnoea.[312,313] Adduction (closure) of the larynx, particularly before lung aeration, may reduce the effectiveness of non-invasive respiratory support.[314]

CPAP and PEEP from birth

If the baby is breathing spontaneously then applying continuous positive airway pressure (CPAP), using either the face mask or where available nasal prongs, will ease the work of breathing and help to prevent alveolar collapse in expiration.[218] Many preterm babies can be stabilised on CPAP at birth without any need for intubation.[315] Suitable CPAP levels are five to eight cm water. In the ventilated baby, airway recruitment can be increased and end-expiratory airway collapse reduced by maintaining positive end expiratory pressure (PEEP). An appropriate starting PEEP is 5 cm water.

Gentle and gradual aeration

If lung expansion and positive pressure ventilation is needed at birth, the aim should be to gently expand the lungs of the baby to gradually maximise gas exchange surface area, to avoid over-distension while at the same time preventing collapse during expiration.

In experiments in preterm lambs, use of large inflation volumes immediately after delivery caused significant damage. This damage was slightly less if surfactant was given before inflation. However, if large tidal volumes, were only used after 10 min of more gentle ventilation much less damage was done.[316] This would suggest that a more gradual approach may be an advantage rather than aiming for rapid achievement of full lung inflation.

Inflation breaths help to establish a resting lung volume, but sustained inflation with breaths longer than 5 s should be avoided; meta-analysis of studies comparing the use of sustained lung inflations (of at least 5 s duration) showed they offer no benefit compared to the standard approach[184] and one of the included studies, the SAIL trial,[185] saw an excess of deaths when using sustained inflations of 15 s in extremely preterm babies.

The fetus copes with its relatively hypoxic environment; its arterial partial pressure of oxygen (PaO_2) is 3.0–3.5 kPa (25–30 mmHg) and in the first few minutes after birth this will increase to 10.5–12.0 kPa (80–90 mmHg). Various researchers have now shown that brief and sudden exposure of the fetus that has existed with its relative hypoxia to high concentrations of inspired oxygen could have detrimental effects.[317,318] For preterm babies a gestation-based approach (Table 9.2) to initial oxygen concentration is used.[31,319]

Table 9.2   Recommended initial oxygen concentrations in newborn preterm infants

Gestation	Starting concentration of oxygen
> 32 weeks	Air
28+0–32+0 weeks	21–30%
< 28+0 weeks	30%

Early saturation monitoring helps to avoid under or over oxygenation, titrate the oxygen concentration according to the saturations using Table 9.3 as a guide and avoiding saturations greater than 95%.

Table 9.3	Acceptable right arm oxygen saturations after birth
Time from birth	Acceptable (25th centile) right arm oxygen saturations
2 min	65%
5 min	85%
10 min	90%

Tidal volume

The lungs of preterm newborn babies are uniquely susceptible to injury because they are structurally immature, surfactant-deficient, fluid-filled and not supported by a stiff chest wall, and significant damage can be caused by even a small number of over-enthusiastic breaths. We can guard against this volume trauma to some extent by limiting the pressure applied to the gas in the airway, but the best way is by limiting the volume change of the lung itself. This implies that the future may lie in measuring and adjusting the tidal volume administered rather than trying to estimate this clinically or via a proxy measurement of pressure.[320]

If it is possible to include devices measuring expired tidal volume into equipment used for stabilising preterm babies at birth, these may be helpful. Exactly what tidal volumes are safe and effective is not yet known but they should probably be approximately 4–8 mL kg^{-1}, which approximates the normal tidal volume of a spontaneously breathing newborn preterm baby receiving CPAP.[321]

Pressure and volume

If you are using a T-piece, start with inflation pressures of 25 cm water, even then it is still possible to inadvertently produce tidal volumes in excess of 10 mL kg^{-1}. If these pressures, applied for 2–3 s, are unsuccessful, higher pressures can be tried. Inflation pressures of up to 30 cm water may be required but should be avoided, if possible, to reduce the risk of lung injury in survivors. Once chest rise is achieved you should consider reducing the pressure. If significant chest expansion is easily seen it is likely that inflation volumes are too great and over-distension of the lung may be occurring.

The best guide as to whether satisfactory lung inflation is being maintained is a sustained increase in the heart rate. If the heart rate has increased satisfactorily then ventilation is probably adequate. Only if the heart rate has not stabilised should you seek to increase the degree of chest expansion. Clinical judgement is unreliable when assessing tidal volume based on chest excursion.[308,322]

If a preterm baby appears to need continued ventilation rather than CPAP, they should be connected to a ventilator as soon as possible and the settings adjusted to avoid excessive tidal volume.

Avoid over-distension of the lungs
Start with pressures of 25 cm water in babies < 32 weeks gestation and use PEEP (5 cm water)
Increase or decrease the pressure according to response

Intubation

Few preterm babies, even those born before 28 weeks gestation, require intubation at birth. Intubation with the correct size tracheal tube can make the ventilation of abnormally stiff lungs easier and will also allow administration of surfactant. Inflation pressures should be delivered in a controlled manner in order to avoid excessive inspiratory volumes, which might risk significant lung injury. Control of inspiratory pressure is most easily achieved using a T-piece system rather than a bag-mask device. Ideally PEEP of 5 cm water should be applied to reduce alveolar collapse in expiration and thus avoid the inevitable shearing forces which occur when collapsed alveoli and small airways are re-expanded.[323]

Some babies will also deliver unexpectedly outside the labour ward where the attendant may not only be inexperienced at intubation, but also have minimal equipment. It is safer to avoid intubation in such circumstances.[324] The normal algorithm should be followed, paying particular attention to drying the baby and keeping the baby covered and warm or placing into a polythene bag and placed next to the mother's skin, and instituting good airway control and mask ventilation if necessary.

Surfactant therapy

For babies less than 30 weeks gestation, there is a significant risk of Respiratory Distress Syndrome (RDS) and evidence, in intubated babies, that early prophylactic use of surfactant has advantages over rescue treatment.[325] Any baby of 30 weeks or less who has a tracheal tube placed should almost certainly receive surfactant with the aim of facilitating early extubation to CPAP support.

Primary use of CPAP, with or without the use of surfactant, can reduce the number of preterm babies needing long-term ventilation. It is possible to administer surfactant without intubation; the Less Invasive Surfactant Administration (LISA) involves passing a small catheter through the vocal cords whilst maintaining nasal CPAP.[326] Surfactant may also be given via a laryngeal mask.[327]

Avoid both hyperoxaemia and hypoxia

Stabilisation or resuscitation of significantly preterm babies (32 weeks or less) may be started with air or supplemental oxygen up to 30% (see Table 9.2). Subsequently oxygen concentration should be guided by pulse oximetry.

Using a pulse oximeter to monitor both heart rate and oxygen saturation in these babies from birth makes stabilisation much easier (Appendix 3). Exposing babies at birth to high concentrations of oxygen can have significant adverse longer-term effects.[318,328] The study reporting normal values for right arm (pre-ductal) oxygen saturation levels in the first minutes after birth from over 450 babies contained data from only 39 babies born before 32 weeks gestation.[134] The 25th centile saturation levels in these preterm babies was very slightly lower than the same centile constructed from the data from all the babies in the study. Table 9.3 is the same as that in Chapter 5 and shows the 25th centile values for all the babies in the study.

For practical purposes the same values of 'acceptable' oxygen saturation can be used for both term and preterm infants. Remember, these saturation levels are deemed 'acceptable' in the sense that babies exhibiting these levels or higher probably do not need any supplemental oxygen. However, babies whose saturation levels are significantly lower might warrant careful supplementation.

Saturations of < 80% at 5 min should prompt a gradual increase in supplemental oxygen, titrated to reliable pulse oximeter saturation reading, to achieve acceptable pre-ductal saturations. For those babies < 32 weeks gestation the target should be to avoid an oxygen saturation below 80% and/or bradycardia at 5 minutes of age. Both are associated with poor outcome.[213]

And the rare preterm baby who actually needs resuscitation?

Preterm babies between 32+0 and 36+6 weeks should be resuscitated using the standard NLS approach.

For preterm babies born before 32+0 weeks requiring resuscitation, you should also follow the standard NLS approach but modify the following components:

- **Thermal care** – babies should be placed in a polythene bag under a radiant heater immediately.
- **Inspiratory pressures** – start with lower inflation pressures of 25 cm water.
- **Expiratory pressures** – use a PEEP of 5 cm water.
- **Initial oxygen concentration** – use 21–30% oxygen (see Table 9.2).
- **Early use of oxygen saturation monitoring.**

The presence of bradycardia and hypoxia adds urgency to the need to establish effective ventilation, and the situation is no longer one of encouraging gentle transition. Any hypoxia will continue until effective lung inflation and ventilation is established.

Start with 5 inflation breaths at pressures of 25 cm water with a background PEEP of 5 cm water. If the chest does not rise and the heart rate is not improving, ensure the airway is open and increase ventilation pressures gradually until visible chest expansion is identifiable. Consider reducing ventilation pressures as soon as you achieve an increase in increase in heart rate.

Although preterm infants at risk of RDS may benefit from surfactant replacement, this should not be considered a drug of resuscitation as a bolus of surfactant may briefly compromise ventilation before it becomes more widely distributed.

09: Summary learning

Most preterm babies need support and 'assisted transition' in the minutes after birth rather than resuscitation.

Clamping of the cord should be delayed unless it prevents resuscitation required by the mother or baby.

Polythene bags and overhead warming are the best methods for preventing hypothermia. Consider early temperature monitoring.

Establish oxygen saturation monitoring as soon as you can and adjust the air/oxygen blender to avoid hyperoxia and hypoxia.

If the baby has satisfactory oxygen saturation and heart rate and is making regular breathing attempts try mask or nasal prong CPAP, starting with air to 30% oxygen, depending on the gestation.

If the baby does not breathe, begin inflation breaths using an inspiratory pressure of 25 cm water and PEEP of 5 cm water, start with air to 30% oxygen depending on the gestation.

If the preterm baby does need intubating, consider early use of surfactant.

My key take-home messages from this chapter are:

Birth outside labour ward

The learning outcomes will enable you to:

Understand the practitioner's role in preparing to manage effective resuscitation of the newborn baby in planned or unplanned birth outside the hospital labour ward

Prepare equipment, environment and colleagues to support effective resuscitation of the newborn

Balance the psychological needs of the mother and family, with ensuring the safety of mother and baby through birth and early postnatal period

Appreciate the importance of record keeping around resuscitation of the newborn outside labour ward

Introduction

Birth outside labour ward may be planned or unplanned. Planned home births usually involve low-risk pregnancies in which the birth is 'due to take place after 37 completed weeks to 42 weeks gestation and a normal birth is expected'.[155]

For planned home births, the mother, birth partner and all healthcare individuals can collaborate and agree details concerning who will attend the birth, when and how they will be called, what equipment will be needed, how it will be obtained, and what the backup arrangements are in case of emergencies. As the need for resuscitation cannot always be predicted, even in a low-risk setting like planned home birth, practitioners must have the knowledge and skills to initiate resuscitation should it be needed.

However, if the birth is unplanned, often none of these arrangements will have been made; in addition, the pregnancy may not be a 'low-risk' pregnancy for either the mother or the baby. It may further be complicated by the baby being preterm.[329] This chapter will aim to cover both situations with suggestions as to how to support and resuscitate the baby. In the majority of births outside hospital, the professional supervising the birth is a midwife. Most deliveries are attended by two midwives; the first attends from the beginning and then calls the second at the end of the first stage. One midwife can then attend to the mother and the second to the baby. If a second midwife is unavailable at the time of delivery, the midwife must be aware of the physical wellbeing of both the mother and the baby.

Planned home births

Planned births outside hospital should be only be offered when there are clear and timely referral and transfer arrangements in place in case of emergencies or complications. The suitability of home births should be discussed in advance with the expectant mother and her partner.

In women with a 'low-risk' second or subsequent pregnancy, a planned home birth is as safe as hospital birth for the baby, and less likely to involve medical intervention to the mother. This is not quite the case for expectant mothers in their first pregnancy where there is a greater risk of adverse perinatal outcome compared to planned delivery in an obstetric unit.[330] It is important, therefore, that mothers planning a home birth are offered an informed choice and that midwives who attend such deliveries are trained in newborn resuscitation.

Commissioners and providers of maternity care should ensure that there are:

- robust protocols in place for transfer of care between settings
- clear local pathways for the continued care of women who are transferred from one setting to another.

Furthermore, in some localities this should also take into consideration the need to cross provider boundaries if the nearest obstetric or neonatal unit (NNU) is closed to admissions or the local midwifery-led unit is full.

All NHS maternity care providers must ensure that community-based facilities have appropriate equipment to provide newborn life support and staff have the skills for initial management and referral. During the antenatal period, the mother and family should have been made aware of the midwifery on-call arrangements, the preparations to be made within the home, what equipment may be required and any transfer arrangements and procedures.

The presence of meconium-stained liquor should prompt the transfer of the mother to hospital before delivery as the meconium may be an indicator of fetal compromise. If there is no time to transfer the mother, then the approach to the baby should be the same as described in Chapter 7.

Environment

Preparing the environment

A suitable area for attending to the baby needs to be identified and prepared in advance. A firm, flat elevated surface area should be cleared and towels made ready.

Close the windows and doors to prevent draughts. Use stand-alone heaters or heated mattress if available. Chose a suitable area for resuscitation, if required, and use warm radiators to heat towels. But be careful not to overheat them; test the temperature against the inner aspect of your forearm. Hot water bottles can also be useful to heat the surface area but should never be put in direct contact with the baby.

Temperature

Maintaining the normal temperature of the baby can be more difficult outside hospital, but it remains equally, if not more important as in a hospital setting. Cover the baby's head with a hat and then, if appropriate, place the baby in direct skin-to-skin contact with the mother, or another warm adult body, under a dry towel or under clothing. If skin-to-skin contact is provided it is vital to observe the newborn baby's airway at all times and the mother needs to be made aware of the importance of this by, for example, avoiding other distractions such as using social media, due to the risks of sudden unexpected postnatal collapse (SUPC).[44,45] Alternatively, the baby should be dried and wrapped in warm towels or clothing. Polythene bags are a further option in both term and preterm babies outside of labour wards when the delivery is unplanned or the baby is ill, however a heat source will also be required.[305,306]

Timing

Use your watch, smartphone or a clock (preferably one that shows seconds as well as hours and minutes) to enable accurate documentation of times.

Equipment

Exactly what equipment should be carried for planned home births is a matter for local decision. A suggested minimum list is available through the Resuscitation Council UK website (www.resus.org.uk).

The choice of equipment is very much a pragmatic one, A self-inflating bag allows the delivery of inflation breaths using room air with the ability to increase the inspired oxygen to different levels; oxygen concentrations of approximately 70% can be achieved by attaching an oxygen supply to the self-inflating bag without its reservoir bag if this can be removed[214,216] and nearly 100% if a reservoir bag is used.[215]

T-piece and blender combinations that allow accurate and controlled delivery of variable pressures and variable oxygen concentrations in a hospital setting are not widely available in a form that is very suitable for a home birth as the additional weight (particularly of the oxygen cylinder) is often prohibitive. Newer T-piece equipment are, however, becoming more portable and may lend itself to being able to deliver variable pressure from portable cylinders.[331]

At birth

If possible, two healthcare professionals, at least one of whom is a registered midwife, need to be present at the birth. Tasks should be allocated depending on the situation and the skills of those available. Detailed discussion of the midwifery and obstetric practicalities are beyond the scope of this text, but physiological management of the third stage is likely to be very appropriate in this situation and will allow for delayed cord clamping (DCC), the benefits of which are outlined in Chapter 6.

It also becomes easier to focus attention on the baby if physiological management of the third stage is used. Active management of the third stage using ergometrine/oxytocin may delay attendance on the baby. The resuscitation of the newborn in the home, as in any other environment, follows the standard algorithm.

Help

Within any locality where home births take place, an agreed system of 'who should be called when' needs to be in place. In most cases, help will be available via an emergency call for a paramedic ambulance, but in more remote areas other means may be used. If the home does not have a landline or mobile phone reception, an alternative form of contact must be arranged.

Transfer

If a baby has needed resuscitation at birth, then transfer to hospital is required following stabilisation. If only one midwife is present, then both the mother and baby should be transferred and not be separated during that transfer unless this is unavoidable. The ambulance staff should be asked to increase the temperature in the ambulance prior to transfer. If the temperature is uncomfortably warm for an adult, it will be about right for the baby.

If the baby is maintaining their airway, they can be transported held close to mother. However, if the baby requires support, special arrangements will be needed. Usual practice is for the baby to be brought to a hospital using a paramedic ambulance. If a decision has been made to bring the baby into hospital whilst still being resuscitated, the stretcher is used as a base to resuscitate the baby; it should be covered with towels and the baby placed on top to continue resuscitation procedures. For any term or near-term baby requiring airway support during transfer, the laryngeal mask offers a more effective means of maintaining airway patency than face mask ventilation whilst in the back of a moving vehicle.[332] The environment should be as warm as possible. Remember to consider the safety of the whole team in this situation.

Unplanned births outside labour ward

Help must be called early; you will almost certainly need it. Unplanned births are more likely to be premature or involving babies or women with health problems. An unplanned birth may occur anywhere an expectant mother might be. The approach to resuscitation is the same anywhere but the availability of equipment, personnel and experience will obviously vary; most unplanned deliveries in the UK will be attended by ambulance service personnel.[333]

Mouth-to-mouth resuscitation (Chapter 7) may be required if the baby is not breathing.

Birth in an ambulance

1. Stop the ambulance

It is not possible to manage a birth safely in a moving ambulance. Ask the crew to stop the ambulance and increase the heating. One of the ambulance crew should make immediate radio contact with ambulance control who can relay the information to the nearest maternity unit or other centre.

2. Mother

Ask the mother to sit upright if possible as this will leave space to deal with the newborn. Leave the cord intact, ideally for at least 60 s, while you assess the baby and the need for resuscitation. Leave the placenta to deliver physiologically after clamping and cutting the cord. Support the mother and do not attempt to deliver the placenta in transit. Observe progress of the third stage of labour and monitor for bleeding.

3. Baby

The baby should be resuscitated, if needed, in the standard manner. Once the baby is safely born, make sure the baby is kept warm, continue to make clinical observations and restart the journey. A baby in good condition can be given to the mother for skin-to-skin contact (Figure 3.1), or else wrapped and held by the mother. Plastic bags can also be useful in this situation.[305,306] The safety aspects of holding a baby in the back of a moving ambulance should be considered.

Record keeping

Clinical records of the birth at home must be maintained in exactly the same way as they are for births in a hospital setting. These records must be continued during the transfer and shared with the receiving team.

10: Summary learning

In any birth outside the hospital setting, take control of the environment and follow the standard NLS algorithm:

- Unplanned out-of-hospital deliveries are generally higher risk than planned ones.

- Consider how to optimise the out-of-hospital birth setting.

- Call for help early, bear in mind this may take longer to arrive in an out-of-hospital setting.

- Dry, warm and cover the baby, consider ambient temperature in an out-of-hospital setting.

- Assess the situation and consider umbilical cord management.

- Open the airway, give inflation breaths.

- Give ventilation breaths and ensure chest rise for 30 s.

- As long as ventilation breaths are effective then give chest compressions if the heart rate remains very slow.

- Continue until help arrives and plan safe transfer to a hospital setting if appropriate.

My key take-home messages from this chapter are:

Post-resuscitation care, prognostication and communication

11

In this chapter

Immediate and later post-resuscitation monitoring and care

Determining the likely cause for requiring resuscitation

The implications of a baby being in primary or secondary apnoea

When to consider therapeutic hypothermia

The prognosis of babies requiring resuscitation

Keeping accurate records and communicating with parents and professional colleagues after a resuscitation

The learning outcomes will enable you to:

Understand the need to:

- assess risk of subsequent physiological problems requiring stabilisation
- transfer to a neonatal unit for further care following significant resuscitation

Describe some of the most common problems which may occur after significant resuscitation

Discuss the use of use of therapeutic hypothermia (cooling) for babies with hypoxic ischaemic encephalopathy (HIE); who can be treated and how and when it should be considered

Understand that good communication is critically important in the support of distressed parents and the healthcare team

Realise that a common theme in external case reviews is a lack of clear documentation and rationale for treatment, so clear note keeping is essential

Introduction

Immediate resuscitation is complete once the baby has adequate ventilation (spontaneous or assisted) and a stable heart rate of more than 100 min^{-1}. However, further stabilisation may be needed to avoid later clinical deterioration following a prolonged resuscitation. This may require transfer to a neonatal unit for high dependency or intensive care.

This chapter summarises the ongoing management of the baby who has required resuscitation at birth, including a summary of prognostic factors and the importance of good communication and record keeping. The reader should be aware that this is not a comprehensive list and the review represents current opinion as well as the evidence where this exists. Most babies who require some resuscitation at birth will quickly stabilise and may remain with their parents. However, some babies, especially if they have required extensive or prolonged resuscitation, will require additional monitoring and intensive care support.

Immediate post-resuscitation care

1. Monitoring return of circulation and breathing

Behaviour during recovery from a hypoxic insult is a guide to the length and severity of the episode and should be monitored and documented carefully. Once the circulation is restored, agonal gasping, occurring every 5–8 s, is almost always the first sign of recovery from terminal apnoea. Ventilation should continue until normal regular breathing is established. Gasping may continue after normal respiratory activity appears. One indicator of the duration and or severity of the hypoxic insult to the central nervous system is the length of time from the return of a normal heart rate to the onset of normal regular respiration (with or without intermittent additional gasps).[123,334]

2. Continued airway support

If intubation has been necessary and extubation is not appropriate, the tracheal tube must have tested positive for exhaled CO_2, be secured, and have equal breath sounds audible on both sides of the chest, before transfer to the neonatal unit. Positive end expiratory pressure (PEEP) should be used. Avoid over-ventilation during transfer and try to avoid both hyperoxaemia and hypocapnia.[335] Consider exogenous surfactant in any intubated and ventilated baby in whom surfactant-deficiency may lead to Respiratory Distress Syndrome (RDS).[336]

Once safely on the NNU, a chest x-ray should be done, and if the tube tip position has been confirmed as satisfactory, any external excess length of tube beyond the point of securing ('dead space') can be removed to allow easier nursing care and optimise ventilation.

3. Location of post-resuscitation care

Once the initial stabilisation phase is over, a care plan is needed which balances the desire to keep the baby with the mother where possible, against the need for close observation and high dependency support in babies at significant risk of post-resuscitation problems.[337]

When making decisions about ongoing post-resuscitation care, consider the following as part of a risk assessment:

- How great were the concerns of maternity staff about fetal wellbeing in labour?
- How is the baby now? What is the tone, heart rate, breathing?
- Do the umbilical cord gases show severe acidosis?
- Was the baby floppy, extremely bradycardic and without any respiratory effort at birth?
- How long did the baby take to respond to resuscitation?
- Were chest compressions used?
- Was gasping seen at any stage?
- Is the baby preterm, small for gestational age or growth restricted?
- Does the baby meet therapeutic hypothermia (cooling) criteria?

Observation is also warranted for babies who are at risk of infection, or from the side effects of maternal medication. Less commonly, babies with prenatally diagnosed disorders may need to be more closely monitored in the period after birth. The level of observation and location (e.g. the neonatal unit, transitional care, postnatal ward) needs to be considered.

4. Remaining with mother

If the decision is that the baby should remain with the mother, a clear plan of management should be documented and should include advice to feed early and specify the need to observe temperature, pulse and respirations on a regular basis. A newborn early warning score chart e.g. the British Association of Perinatal Medicine 'Newborn Early Warning Trigger & Track' ('NEWTT') score chart can be helpful in providing clear guidance on when to seek review and will help to avoid any deterioration being missed.[338,339] The length of the observation period depends on the clinical status and potential underlying problems and can range from several minutes to several hours as babies transition. In most cases, problems with transition resolve fairly quickly after birth, and the period of more intensive observation can be safely concluded without resorting to admission to the neonatal unit.

5. Transfer to the neonatal unit

Continuing observation is necessary for any post-resuscitation baby who continues to have abnormal signs or symptoms, especially if there is a need for ongoing support.

When moving the baby for transfer, they should be kept warm, airway, breathing and circulation should be stable enough to transfer and any intravenous lines secured. Appropriate transport equipment should be used and monitoring should be used during transfer e.g. oxygen saturation and heart rate monitoring. The needs of the parents should be considered, ensuring that they are fully informed of events, the reasons for transfer, where their baby is going and ongoing care.

> Ensure that the baby is wearing their identity bracelets before they leave the delivery area

In any situation, complete the notes as soon as possible. Recording of events during resuscitation is generally inaccurate and poorly documented yet such records are necessary from an ethical, legal, research and quality improvement viewpoint.[125] Record the baby's condition at birth, the resuscitation sequence and the baby's response to that resuscitation. When possible, ensure that an explanation of the sequence of events is given to parents and document what they have been told.

6. Debriefing the team

Whilst the ongoing stabilisation of the baby remains the priority for the clinical team, it is important to acknowledge the huge impact a full resuscitation has on all members of the team. At the earliest opportunity, and ideally on the same shift, once the baby's initial clinical needs have been met and parents updated, a debrief should be arranged. This is discussed in more detail in Chapter 13.

Determining the root cause of the problem

When determining the likely underlying cause(s) of problems encountered it should be remembered that it may be multifactorial. Also, babies with underlying antenatal problems are more likely to undergo a birth process which involve acute or subacute hypoxia.

Acute hypoxia

The prognosis for the term baby subjected to a sudden acute hypoxic insult (e.g. from a cord prolapse or shoulder dystocia) can be very good, provided the episode does not last too long. Occasionally, however, even though the circulation is rapidly and effectively restored, cerebral function may be slow to recover.

The length of time taken for reflex gasping activity to return gives some indication of the magnitude of the cerebral insult. However, the length of time it takes for regular breathing to recover once the circulation is restored is a much more easily recorded event that gives a good indication of the severity of the cerebral insult.

Babies who have not established an adequate respiratory drive by 30 minutes of age are likely to have a significant brain injury.[340] Many healthy survivors show cerebral irritability for a few days and some have fits. Cerebral function monitoring (CFM) using an amplitude-integrated EEG (aEEG) is helpful in assessing if babies meet cooling criteria and may provide evidence of seizure activity.[341]

The prognosis for a preterm baby less than 34 weeks gestation subjected to severe acute hypoxia is more unpredictable. There is a risk of secondary intraventricular haemorrhage or periventricular intracerebral haemorrhage and/or infarction after even a relatively brief severe hypoxic episode, especially in the crucial period immediately before and after birth.

Ultrasound scans may not be accurate in establishing the degree of brain injury, although babies with major lesions on cerebral ultrasound are at risk of severe developmental delay. However, the correlation between the initial appearances and eventual outcome may not be sufficiently sensitive to be singularly predictive of poor outcome. Consequently, they may not be helpful in decisions regarding appropriate continuation of intensive care. Similarly, normal scans are not reassuring if the clinical picture suggests a poor prognosis. MRI at term is more helpful.

Chronic intrauterine hypoxia

Chronic intrauterine hypoxia can lead to aspiration of vernix or meconium deep into the lung, put the cardiac musculature under severe strain, promote hypertrophy of muscle within pulmonary arterioles, or cause significant renal damage.[342] It can cause serious cerebral ischaemia or haemorrhage, especially in the preterm baby. In the term baby, ischaemia can cause secondary cerebral oedema after a short, and deceptively encouraging, latent period.

Severe chronic intrauterine hypoxia appears to be more damaging than acute severe hypoxia. The analogy is that sudden severe hypoxia stops the 'engine' abruptly whereas chronic fuel starvation, associated with severe chronic intrauterine hypoxia, 'wrecks the machinery' before the 'engine' finally fails. This chronic intrauterine hypoxia risks secondary cerebral oedema and apoptosis and is associated with reperfusion injury. This may cause more damage than the original period of hypoxia itself. In addition, although the fetal heart (with a large reserve of glycogen) is remarkably resistant to acute hypoxic stress, chronic intrauterine hypoxia may damage the myocardium resulting in low cardiac output.[343] This has secondary consequences for other organs particularly the kidney, which may develop 'pre-renal' failure due to poor perfusion, or acute tubular necrosis, if that hypoperfusion has been severe.

An amplitude-integrated EEG (aEEG), or cerebral function monitor (CFM) can be helpful, and is available in many neonatal units. An electroencephalogram (EEG) can be helpful but requires expert interpretation to be useful. Recent large doses of anticonvulsants will make interpretation even more difficult. Long-term prognosis depends largely on the depth of the post-hypoxic coma, the extent of any secondary cerebral oedema, and the severity and persistence of any seizure activity.

The extent of cerebral injury becomes more apparent following assessment over 36–48 hours following an acute hypoxic insult. A mild short-lasting state of hyper-excitability usually carries a good prognosis even if there is seizure activity, but prolonged abnormal neurology can be associated with more severe developmental delay. Being able to enterally feed successfully at a week of age is a good prognostic marker.[344]

A quarter of babies with Grade 2 Hypoxic Ischaemic Encephalopathy (HIE), according to the modified classification of Sarnat and Sarnat (summarised in Appendix 1), suffer moderate developmental delay. The prognosis is worse if there are seizures. Most babies who are flaccid and stuporose (Grade 3 HIE) will not survive, and if they do survive risk moderate to severe developmental delay.[345]

Discriminating between primary and terminal apnoea

There is no instant way of predicting if a baby is in primary apnoea and, therefore, merely needs a clear airway, or in terminal apnoea and needing active help. An Apgar score is frequently retrospective (and subjective) and indicates how unresponsive the baby is (which in turn may be due to shock, maternal sedation or simply immaturity rather than hypoxia). A cord pH only quantifies acidosis at that moment.

Observation of the sequence of events during recovery will provide more information regarding cause of unresponsiveness. One measure of the anoxic insult to the central nervous system is the length of time from the return of a normal heart rate to the onset of normal regular respiration (with or without intermittent additional gasps).[63]

As oxygen returns to the brain, the various control centres recover. As the baby responds it will exhibit changes in behaviour in reverse order to that shown as it deteriorated, which should help to determine how far the baby had deteriorated. Babies who have been in terminal apnoea do not cough or gasp until the circulation is restored and usually exhibit a period of gasping before the onset of normal breathing movements.[123]

Umbilical cord blood gases

If there are concerns that the baby has been significantly compromised, cord blood should be taken for measurement of pH, base deficit and lactate, ideally from an umbilical artery as well as from the umbilical vein (i.e. a 'paired' blood gas).[346-349] Both arterial and venous umbilical cord blood gas status is easily determined if two clamps are put on a 10 cm segment of the cord around a minute after birth and the isolated portion put aside. Ideally these should be sampled and processed within 10 minutes. Blood pH estimation in samples from double-clamped vessels is reliable for up to 60 minutes but measurements of lactate are only reliable if analysed within 20 minutes.[349]

Umbilical cord gases can still be obtained after delayed cord clamping, however there are some suggestions that various parameters can change significantly during the period when the cord remains unclamped (see Appendix A).

Labelling the placenta for later examination

Detailed examination of the placenta, including a histological examination, may provide vital evidence regarding the reason why a baby required resuscitation at birth. The placenta should be labelled and histopathological examination requested. Placental pathological diagnoses can suggest aetiologies such as metabolic disorders, adverse growth events and infections as well as an alternative explanation for neonatal encephalopathy other than acute intrapartum hypoxia.[351]

Kleihauer test

If a baby is born with significant anaemia, feto-maternal haemorrhage should be considered as a differential diagnosis. It is important to request that a sample of blood is taken from the mother and a Kleihauer test requested (which tests for evidence of feto-maternal bleeding). The Kleihauer (sometimes called Kleihauer-Betke) test detects fetal cells, which contain HbF, in the maternal blood.[352] In addition to simply detecting feto-maternal haemorrhage, a Kleihauer test may be able to estimate the volume of the haemorrhage.

Sepsis

Sepsis should always be considered as a possible underlying cause for, and may be the primary reason for, perinatal compromise. If this is a possibility, blood cultures should be taken and treatment commenced within 1 hour of consideration of this diagnosis.[353] The placenta should be sent for later histological examination as above.

Therapeutic hypothermia (cooling)

Perinatal hypoxia severe enough to cause HIE is estimated to occur in approximately 1–6 per 1000 births.[354] HIE and its sequelae presents a major burden for the individual, the family and for society.[355]

Whilst the primary hypoxic brain injury cannot be undone, secondary brain damage, due to cellular apoptosis and the release of excitatory amino acids, occurs. Hypothermia reduces the metabolic rate of the body, including the brain, reducing the secondary brain damage, and resulting in improved neurological outcomes in babies with moderate HIE.

Following the results of three randomised controlled trials, including the UK total body cooling (TOBY) trial,[356] it was confirmed that 72 hours of cooling to a core temperature of 33–34°C, started within six hours of birth, reduces death and disability at 18 months of age. Following a meta-analysis of these data[61] the treatment was recommended by the National Institute for Health and Care Excellence (NICE)[357] and is supported by the British Association of Perinatal Medicine (BAPM).[358]

Therapeutic hypothermia reduces mortality without increasing major disability in survivors[359] and is now a standard of care for infants with moderately severe HIE; it is, however, an intervention that should begin only after any resuscitation. There is no evidence that therapeutic hypothermia started before management of airway, breathing and circulation is effective, and if started inappropriately, could be harmful. Once ABCD have been dealt with, and there is a high suspicion of a hypoxic insult, then therapeutic hypothermia can be considered.

Hyperthermia (≥ 38.0°C) should be avoided as it worsens the brain injury following a hypoxic insult.[360]

When to initiate therapeutic hypothermia

In the UK, the criteria for deciding which babies to treat with therapeutic hypothermia have largely been adopted, with minor local variations, from those used in the TOBY trial.[356] These state that babies in the following categories may be considered for treatment:

- ≥ 36+0 weeks completed gestation and admitted to the neonatal unit
- required resuscitation at birth
- develop seizures or moderate or severe encephalopathy after resuscitation.

The baby should be assessed against, and meet, three criteria: at least one 'A' criterion indicating significant perinatal hypoxia-ischaemia, fulfil 'B' criteria representing the presence of significant neonatal encephalopathy, and at least one 'C' criteria showing seizures or abnormal background activity on aEEG. In order to assess all three criteria means that the baby should have reached the NNU; cooling should not be started prior to this assessment.

Babies who meet criteria A are then assessed to see whether they meet the neurological abnormality entry criteria (criteria B). NOTE: these criteria are only evident after a resuscitation.

If a baby meets both Criteria A and B then they should be assessed using an aEEG to assess whether they meet Criteria C.

When cooling is initiated (either active or passive), this should be done in accordance with the network guidelines and local care pathways and after discussion with their designated network neonatal intensive care unit (NICU). Continuous temperature monitoring should in place using a rectal temperature probe.

Some neonatal networks have agreed extended inclusion and exclusion criteria and the BAPM framework[358] includes guidance in the use of therapeutic hypothermia in following groups of babies who do not fit the TOBY clinical trial criteria:

Babies identified after 6 hours but before 24-hours of age

There is little data to support or refute the use of hypothermia in these babies and every effort should be to identify and diagnose moderate to severe HIE in a timely fashion. In the absence of other treatments, clinicians may consider offering therapeutic hypothermia to this group of babies.

Babies less than 36 weeks gestation

There are currently no randomised controlled trial data to support use in these babies. Therapeutic hypothermia might be considered after a detailed discussion with the parents including explaining the risks (which potentially may be greater in late preterm babies and the lack of evidence suggesting benefit. A second opinion from an experienced consultant is recognised as good practice in this situation.

Criteria A

Infants who fall into the above groups and who are admitted to the neonatal unit meet criteria A if they have at least one of the following:

- Apgar score of ≤ 5 at 10 minutes after birth
- continued need for resuscitation, including tracheal or mask ventilation, at 10 min after birth*
- acidosis within 60 min of birth (defined as any occurrence of umbilical cord, arterial or capillary pH < 7.00)
- base deficit ≥ 16 mmol L^{-1} in umbilical cord or any blood sample (arterial, venous or capillary) within 60 minutes of birth.

* NOTE: The term 'continued need for resuscitation including mask or tracheal ventilation' refers only to those babies receiving positive pressure ventilation and does not include those babies who are receiving PEEP or CPAP.

Criteria B

Moderate to severe encephalopathy, consisting of altered state of consciousness (lethargy, stupor or coma) AND at least one of the following:

- hypotonia
- abnormal reflexes including oculomotor or pupillary abnormalities
- absent or weak suck.

Criteria C

At least 30 min duration of aEEG recording that shows abnormal background aEEG activity or seizures. There must be one of the following:

- normal background with some seizure activity
- moderately abnormal activity
- suppressed activity
- continuous seizure activity.

Sudden Unexpected Postnatal Collapse (SUPC)

There are some similarities between SUPC and HIE due to perinatal hypoxia providing circumstantial evidence that therapeutic hypothermia might be of benefit. It is important to remember that SUPC has many causes and some of these may be adversely affected by cooling. The BAPM framework recommends that every effort is taken to understand any underlying reasons for collapse before starting therapeutic hypothermia. The decision to cool should be explained to the baby's parents along with an explanation of the potential risks and benefits.

Mild neonatal encephalopathy

There are currently no trial data to support the use of therapeutic hypothermia in this group and it is not to be recommended.

Passive cooling

Once airway, breathing and circulation have been stabilised and a decision has been made to offer cooling, if equipment for active cooling is not available, passive cooling can be started. Then arrangements are made to transfer the baby to a cooling centre. Passive cooling requires monitoring of rectal temperature but its use helps to avoid delays in starting treatment that would otherwise occur.[361]

Other aspects of post-resuscitation care

A number of complications may occur after an anoxic insult. Though they may occur after a profound but acute insult, they are much more common after a less profound but prolonged insult. Almost all babies who qualify for therapeutic hypothermia will show some evidence of dysfunction in one or more other body systems. The following summarises these disturbances.

Respiratory depression

Some babies may need continuing ventilation following a hypoxic insult. Blood gases will need to be monitored and transfer to an intensive care unit will need to be arranged.

Beware over-ventilation. Respiratory acidosis can be treated by increasing ventilatory support. However, it is easy to over ventilate a baby with normal lungs, and important to avoid hypocapnia and hyperoxaemia. Reducing the $PaCO_2$ below 4 kPa reduces cerebral perfusion and is strongly associated with neurological damage.[335,362] There is also evidence that hyperoxaemia is also associated with increased damage, especially if combined with hypocapnia.[363]

Continuous monitoring of oxygenation is important. Persistent pulmonary hypertension of the newborn (PPHN), with blood bypassing the lung through the foramen ovale and/or ductus arteriosus, can rapidly become a serious problem if not detected and treated promptly. Monitoring pre- and post-ductal oxygen saturations is very useful in the initial assessment of PPHN with a difference of 5% or more being significant. Appropriate ventilation and oxygenation may reduce the likelihood of this occurring. Early accurate diagnosis and treatment of this problem can be helped by echocardiographic investigation.

Cardiac function

A transient post-hypoxic myocardial dysfunction may commonly cause hypotension and blood pressure monitoring is essential. Whilst maintaining circulating volume is important, if myocardial function is compromised, treating any hypotension with more than one bolus of fluid may be detrimental (i.e. you should consider inotropic support rather than fluid boluses). Echocardiographic assessment of cardiac function (functional echocardiography), if available, should be used to guide appropriate use of inotropic support.

Metabolic acidosis

Virtually all babies who have been in terminal apnoea will have a degree of metabolic acidosis. When managing this consider:

- Once airway and breathing have been successfully managed and the circulation restored, the metabolic acidosis will usually resolve spontaneously over a few hours
- Bicarbonate is sometimes used during CPR but is rarely required in post-resuscitation management
- Situations where bicarbonate may be used include:
  - very immature babies as a pH of < 7.20 inhibits surfactant
  - persistent pulmonary hypotension
  - severe metabolic acidosis combined with hypotension refractory to inotropes
- If bicarbonate corrections are used then slow partial corrections may be given.

Renal function monitoring

Renal function is often impaired following significant intrapartum hypoxia. Total fluid intake should be restricted to a minimum (40–60 mL kg^{-1} per day) until renal function recovers.

Avoid further damage

Nephrotoxic drugs should be avoided or if they must be used, dosing should be adjusted.

Urine output

Monitor closely. Urine may be present in the bladder at the time of the insult and so initial urine output may be normal.

Weight

Increasing weight can be an indicator of fluid retention. Regularly weighing the baby is useful.

Sodium

Monitor serum sodium closely for hyponatraemia. Assess whether it is due to:

a) oliguria and water retention

b) cellular damage causing sodium redistribution within the body

c) renal loss of sodium, before attempting treatment.

Glucose

Babies undergoing extensive resuscitation become hypoglycaemic.[291] A blood glucose less than 2.6 mmol L^{-1} was seen in a quarter of the babies reported to the national TOBY study registry.[292] Therefore after successful resuscitation, formal steps should be taken to prevent both hypoglycaemia and hyperglycaemia. An intravenous glucose infusion should be considered soon after resuscitation with the goal of avoiding hypoglycaemia.

Efforts should be made to maintain serum glucose in the normal range because in babies with HIE an abnormal early postnatal glycaemic profile (i.e. hypoglycaemia, hyperglycaemia or labile blood glucose) is associated with a distinct and worse pattern of brain injury on MRI compared to HIE alone.[294]

Medications

The combination of impaired renal and hepatic function can adversely impact on the metabolism of many drugs used in the baby recovering from a hypoxic insult. In addition, therapeutic hypothermia may further slow the metabolism of many of the drugs that are metabolised by liver enzymes and dose adjustments may be needed both during the hypothermia and re-warming periods.[364]

Seizures

Seizures commonly occur in the first few hours after a hypoxic insult. They can be subtle and easily missed. Use of a CFM can help clarify whether a baby's movements represent seizure activity. A commonly used first line treatment for neonatal seizures is phenobarbital. At higher doses this can cause respiratory depression. Prolonged seizures may represent a more severe brain injury but it is important to consider hypoglycaemia and electrolyte imbalances as possible, correctable causes.

Palliative care

Some babies that have required extensive resuscitation may have their care reorientated to palliative care on NNU in light of additional information that emerges (e.g. CFM monitoring, refractory hypotension) about their overall clinical condition.

Record keeping

Accurate and comprehensive records are crucial, particularly in resuscitation at birth, because records may be carefully scrutinised years later in medico-legal cases.[365] Multiple national reviews and investigations into neonatal death have shown peripartum note keeping is often a poor standard, lacking rationale for actions, and inaccurate in recording of actions taken.[366-368]

Getting someone not involved in the actual resuscitation to act as a scribe and document things that are communicated to them (e.g. the heart rate) allows for contemporary documentation of important events however even this method will result in some errors.[369] Such contemporaneous notes made during the resuscitation should be included in the medical records. Any baby in whom resuscitation is attempted should have their own set of notes. This is imperative if there were signs of life at any stage. Both the NMC[370] and the GMC[371] stress the important in making notes that are clear, accurate and legible. Records should be made at the same time as the events you are recording or as soon as possible afterwards.

A template or proforma may be useful; however, there are no consensus recommendations on how to document meaningful events or what to include on such templates.[125]

Facts not opinions

Accurate written record should document all that happened as soon as possible after an event. Words used in such a record should be carefully considered and it should be remembered that these could be used in a court of law. The records may assume considerable medico-legal importance in later years. You should avoid using subjective medical terms such as those reported by one study of records; 'low heart rate', 'pink' or 'looking bad' as these are open to interpretation in a number of ways.[366] The term 'flat baby' is particularly unhelpful whether spoken or written. Fact must be distinguished from opinion, and the appropriateness of any adjective should be carefully considered. What was seen and done should be recorded and there must be no assumptions made as to causation. The team debriefing can be used to ensure that all aspects of the resuscitation are captured in the written record.

Facts relating to the birth (e.g. fetal bradycardia, non-reassuring cardiotocograph (CTG) trace, low scalp pH) should be noted. The time of every event should be noted as accurately as possible. Words such as 'asphyxia' and 'fetal distress' should not be used as they are impossible to define in this context. Any reference to the obstetric handling of the case should be purely factual.

Useful things to record

After any resuscitation the following information should be recorded:

- when you were called, by whom, and why
- the time you arrived, who else was there, and the condition of the baby on your arrival
- what you did, when you did it, and the timing and details of any response from the baby. Recording these in sequence is helpful
- whether the baby was floppy at birth
- the baby's heart rate at birth and when it first became fast (i.e. exceeded 100 min^{-1})
- the time when you were first certain that the lungs had been successfully inflated
- whether gasping respiration preceded the onset of rhythmical breathing, when gasping started and how long it lasted
- when the baby started to breathe evenly, regularly and effectively 30–60 min^{-1} (even if gasping is still occurring intermittently)
- if you have used a saturation monitor it is helpful to note the initial reading of both the heart rate and saturations and how these changed with your actions
- the date and time of writing your entry followed by your name, your role and grade, your signature and your professional registration number.

Communication after resuscitation

Communication with other professionals

The obstetrician and midwife responsible for the mother's care should also be informed in a timely manner. Conversations should be documented carefully and should include details of the persons concerned, the content of the exchange and the date and time. At discharge relevant antenatal or postnatal diagnoses should be shared with the General Practitioner, community midwife, health visitor and other members of the primary health care team.

Communication with parents

It is important to remember that the parents are the people to whom all information about their baby should be primarily directed. Ideally the information should be shared with both parents together and only with their explicit permission should information be given to others. Very occasionally circumstances may arise where information has to be shared with other family members first but this will be a very rare event. The reasons for this must be documented.

The birth of a baby is an exceptionally important event for parents and they will be extremely anxious if their baby receives any resuscitation at birth. Always speak to the parents as soon as possible; before birth if circumstances allow and it is thought that resuscitation is likely to be needed (Chapter 6). They will assume the worst even if their baby was only on the resuscitaire for a few minutes. Parents often fear that any baby receiving resuscitation is likely to be 'brain-damaged'. Let them see, touch and hold their baby even if the baby is going to the neonatal unit. However, don't let the baby get cold or hypoxic in the process.

Information given to parents or other family members about the baby and any possible outcomes should be objective and should avoid prejudging care. In particular, the person responsible for resuscitation is not usually in a position to make an informed comment on the management of the pregnancy or labour and delivery. This should be left for midwifery and obstetric staff to deal with. Any discussions with parents should be documented.

Stressful situations can inhibit the retention of information and the use of jargon may further complicate the situation. Check the parents' understanding of the information you have given them by asking them to explain what they think you mean. It is the job of professionals to explain effectively. Good communication helps avoid confusion, complaints and litigation.

Language or other communication barriers

Some parents may have difficulties with communication because of disability or language problems. In these situations, interpreters may have to be used. Using other family members to translate important information is generally bad practice as they may not understand the information they are being asked to give, they may translate the information inaccurately and you risk breaching patient confidentiality. Any information communicated to the parents should be clearly documented and this record should include a note of the parents' reaction to the information and any questions that they ask.

Communicating the decision not to offer life-sustaining treatment

When a decision is made not to resuscitate a baby, the parents should be part of the decision-making process and be in agreement with a plan of management. The reasons for the decision should be documented, along with a record of the discussion with the parents and their reaction. The RCUK ReSPECT form can be a helpful document in situations where resuscitation may be limited or not carried out. In Scotland, a Children and Young People Acute Deterioration Management (CYPADM) form may be more familiar, particularly if palliative or comfort care may take place in the parents' home or a hospice.

11: Summary learning

A baby who has been resuscitated is at risk of further deterioration and post-resuscitation plans should take this into consideration.

Placental pathology and blood tests from mother may help in finding the underlying cause of the baby's problems.

If sepsis is considered, antibiotics should be administered within one hour.

If a baby is not admitted to a neonatal unit, there should be a clear plan for further observation and review.

A baby admitted to the neonatal unit after prolonged resuscitation should have vital signs and biochemistry monitored with appropriate interventions to maintain stability.

Following initial resuscitation, therapeutic hypothermia (cooling) should be considered in babies who meet cooling criteria.

Parents and other professionals should be communicated with clearly and appropriately. Details of what is said to the family and when must be clearly documented in the clinical records.

Clinical records should be clear, detailed, factual, legible, timed, dated and signed.

My key take-home messages from this chapter are:

Babies who do not respond

In this chapter

Common reasons for failure to respond to resuscitative efforts and ways to address these

When to consider stopping resuscitative efforts

Which situations might resuscitation be inappropriate

The legal definitions of live birth and stillbirth

The learning outcomes will enable you to:

Discuss the possible reasons why a baby might not respond to the standard approach

Describe the techniques that might be used to treat these unusual cases

Understand when it may be appropriate to stop resuscitation or inappropriate to start

Considerations when a baby's heart rate doesn't respond after the standard approach

A   B   C   D

The commonest reason for a baby's heart rate failing to improve is inadequate management of airway and breathing.

When a baby's heart rate doesn't respond and you have not seen the chest move, make sure to check:

- Is the baby's head in the neutral position?
- Do you need to reapply the face mask to improve the seal?
- Do you need a second person's help with the airway?
- Do you need jaw thrust?
- Are you using a 2–3 s inflation time?

If all of these are being achieved, consider:

- Is there an obstruction in the airway? (laryngoscope and suction)
- Is an airway needed (either laryngeal mask or oropharyngeal airway)?
- Intubation
- Increasing the inspiratory pressure in increments of 2–5 cm water?

If you have not already done so, call for help.

If the standard NLS approach noted above does not improve the baby's heart rate consider the following:

- Tracheal blockage
- Pneumothorax
- Stiff (poorly compliant) lungs
- Hypovolaemia and blood loss
- Reasons for persistent cyanosis (the baby who remains blue)
- Respiratory depression due to maternal opiates in labour
- Hydrops fetalis.

Material blocking the trachea

Lumps of vernix, blood clot, thick mucus or particulate meconium, if large enough, can obstruct the trachea when they have been inhaled. Any such inhalation will almost always have occurred as the result of gasping before or during delivery.

If, using the standard NLS approach outlined previously, you cannot inflate the lungs despite using a well-fitting mask, consider the possibility of impacted debris in the trachea, particularly if there has been a history of meconium-stained liquor. It is important to remember that meconium is not the only cause of tracheal obstruction.

Tracheal intubation for suctioning should be considered where there is no increase in heart rate and no chest movement with mask ventilation.[18,31,372] If you are not trained to intubate, look into the mouth with a laryngoscope and ensure that the oropharynx is clear, consider whether airway adjuncts such as a laryngeal mask may help. At this point, consider the use of either higher inflation pressures or longer inflation times aiming to get some air into the airway pending the arrival of someone who can intubate. After intubation the tracheal tube should be connected to a suitable adaptor (Figure 7.15 in Chapter 7) to convert it to a 'suction catheter'. Although such adaptors are loosely called 'meconium aspirators' they are useful in clearing the trachea of any particulate matter, not just meconium.

Pneumothorax

If care is taken to limit the inflation pressure used, then pneumothorax is a rare cause of problems at birth. It is not always necessary to drain a pneumothorax in the delivery room, and directly aspirating the chest with a syringe and butterfly needle on the faint suspicion of a pneumothorax may well produce one. There may be antenatal information available to suggest that a pneumothorax is more likely to occur during the course of resuscitation (e.g. if the baby is known to have pulmonary hypoplasia on antenatal scans).

In the very rare situation of a tension pneumothorax, suggested by a cyanosed baby, with bradycardia, who does not respond to ventilation and who has reduced breath sounds on one side, more urgent drainage on labour ward may be needed using needle thoracocentesis (Appendix 2).

If possible, it is best to transfer the baby to the neonatal unit, and if stability permits, confirm the diagnosis by examination with a 'cold-light' or by X-ray before treatment.

Stiff lungs

In some cases, the lungs may be unusually stiff (non-compliant). This might occur in situations where severe oligohydramnios or anhydramnios has led to pulmonary hypoplasia. In these cases, despite the manoeuvres discussed previously, it may not be possible to adequately inflate the lungs and oxygenate the baby. If the clinical situation suggests that stiff lungs may be a contributory factor, and you are confident that the airway is open, it may be worth considering increasing the peak inflation pressure. A good mask seal is important if the benefits of these higher pressures are to be seen, but intubation (or using a laryngeal mask if you cannot intubate) may be better to reduce any leak.

> In a baby whose heart rate is not improving and whose chest does not rise with inflation breaths following additional airway opening manoeuvres (e.g. two-person jaw thrust, laryngeal mask), consider increasing the inspiratory pressure (in increments of 2–5 cm water) and/or the duration of the inflation breaths (e.g. 3–4 s).

This initial period of increased pressure may be sufficient to exceed the higher critical opening pressure of the stiffer lung and enable lung inflation to occur. Once inflated, the pressures required to continue with ventilatory support may be lower. Chest rise may be a guide but if suitable equipment is available, you should measure the tidal volumes to guide you to the pressures required and be prepared to reduce the pressures as soon as possible. There is an increased risk of air leak/pneumothorax with such stiffer lungs, especially when using higher pressures.

The baby who is pale, shocked or hypovolaemic

If chest wall movement has been confirmed and the heart rate does not respond after 30 s of ventilation breaths, chest compressions should be commenced.

While most resuscitation situations will only require one or two cycles of chest compressions to move oxygenated blood back to the heart to improve heart rate, some infants will have a persistent bradycardia despite subsequent intravenous drug administration. In this situation, hypovolaemia should be suspected. In some situations, the obstetric team may be able to provide information before or during delivery that raises the index of suspicion of hypovolaemia earlier in resuscitation.

Hypovolaemic shock at delivery is rare and results from acute, peripartum blood loss. It can occur with placental abruption, or after acute feto-maternal bleeding. Cutting through an anterior placenta during caesarean section can cause fetal blood loss. A ruptured placental vessel (vasa praevia) can easily be missed, as can blood loss into the baby's own abdominal cavity from trauma to the spleen or liver. Partial umbilical cord occlusion may obstruct blood flow through the umbilical vein but not the umbilical arteries (where the blood is at higher pressure) resulting in blood reaching the placenta but failing to return to the baby.[120] A similar problem may follow shoulder dystocia.

Treatment of hypovolaemia involves passing an umbilical venous catheter (if not already done) or if this is not possible an intra-osseus needle. Volume replacement can initially be provided with 10 mL kg^{-1} of 0.9% sodium chloride. A further 10 mL kg^{-1} may be given but excessive amounts of fluid should be avoided. Similarly, O rhesus (D) negative blood may be given; later, 20–40 mL kg^{-1} of blood may be required.

If blood loss is known to be the cause of the baby's condition then, ideally, emergency unmatched O Rhesus (D) negative blood should be used. This should be readily available from a locally agreed central location (e.g. labour ward, main theatre or the emergency department). Sometimes further blood transfusions are needed in the post-resuscitation phase and this can be assessed by watching for a progressive fall in haematocrit or haemoglobin.

The baby who remains blue

If the baby remains blue beyond the first 5–10 min and after the chest is moving but has an acceptable heart rate, you should ensure airway patency, that the chest continues to move and that you have turned the oxygen concentration up. Keep ventilating and call for help. Use a pulse oximeter to check the pre-ductal oxygen saturation if not already applied. Consider using a second oximeter, if available, to simultaneously check the post-ductal oxygen saturation, a difference of ≥ 3% between pre- and post-ductal saturations raises the possibility that you are dealing with a cardiac problem.[373]

Other causes of continued cyanosis in a normal looking term baby are very rare. They include congenital pneumonia or an undiagnosed diaphragmatic hernia. It is rare for congenital cyanotic heart disease to be obvious this early, though some cyanosis can be present from birth. Duskiness can be the first sign of persistent pulmonary hypertension, which can easily spiral rapidly out of control if not recognised and treated quickly.

In the resuscitation situation, a persistent low saturation should be treated with 100% oxygen. You will need to transfer the baby to the neonatal unit in order to investigate the cause for the low saturations further. If a cardiac cause is suspected, seek paediatric cardiology advice as accepting lower oxygen saturations may be appropriate and other clinical management measures may be needed.

Although there are concerns that high concentrations of oxygen might promote closure of the arterial duct, most babies who remain cyanosed will receive 100% oxygen until they can be further assessed in the neonatal unit. It is probably better to accept a temporary exposure to 100% oxygen in such cases than to delay transfer.

> Continued cyanosis and low oxygen saturations require immediate investigation and senior help.

Opiates and naloxone

Babies affected by opiates given to the mother usually cry at birth, but may become apnoeic when wrapped up warm and comfortable a few minutes later.[374] The baby most at risk is one whose mother has had repeated doses of opiates less than three hours apart (the adult half-life), who has had intravenous (IV) rather than intramuscular (IM) doses, or who has received the drug less than 2–3 hours before delivery. If a baby is apnoeic secondary to maternal opiates the priority is for lung aeration and subsequent ventilation. Only when the airway is secure, lung aeration has been achieved, the baby is ventilated and heart rate is normal, should naloxone treatment be considered. Naloxone is not an emergency drug and is not given during resuscitation but rather once the baby is stable from a cardiovascular perspective but remains apnoeic due to maternal opiate administration.

Babies who are apnoeic secondary to maternal opiates should, once their airway (A), breathing (B) and circulation (C) have been addressed, be given 200 micrograms of intramuscular (IM) naloxone (0.5 mL of the standard 400 microgram mL ampoule).

Smaller doses of naloxone, usually given intravenously, are not advised as they wear off quickly and potentially resulting in a return of the baby's opiate-related respiratory depression. This is insufficient to counter the effect of pethidine, for example, which can last for more than 24 hour in the exposed newborn baby. Narcotics accumulate progressively in the unborn baby after administration to the mother.

Hydrops fetalis

Hydrops fetalis is usually diagnosed by antenatal ultrasound, although it may rarely be an unexpected finding at delivery in which case it should prompt an immediate call for senior assistance (a 2222 call may be appropriate). It is a condition in the fetus characterised by an accumulation of fluid, or oedema, in at least two fetal compartments (e.g. the pleural, pericardial or peritoneal cavities and/or the skin). Being aware of the diagnosis can allow the neonatal team useful opportunity to prepare a strategy for resuscitating the baby with hydrops in advance of delivery (see Chapter 6).

The baby will be pale and bloated with generalised oedema, ascites and pleural effusions. A laryngeal mask airway can be useful if higher pressures are necessary and you cannot intubate. If higher pressures do not work, drainage of pleural effusions should then be considered to optimise lung aeration. Pleural effusions only occasionally interfere with lung aeration. It may be necessary to drain the abdominal ascites (from the left iliac fossa, to avoid damage to an enlarged liver or spleen) and apply an airway pressure of more than 30 cm water in order to achieve better diaphragmatic movement and lung aeration.

Ascitic or pleural fluid is best drained with a relatively wide bore needle or cannula (e.g. 20 gauge). In the very rare event that volume is required following ascitic or pleural fluid drainage, use 0.9% sodium chloride.

When should you stop resuscitation?

In the baby with no heart rate at birth, the longer it takes for a return of spontaneous circulation the higher the risk of death and, amongst survivors, severe neurodevelopmental impairment. There is, however, considerable case-by-case variation.[375-377]

Current guidance is to continue resuscitation until at least 20 minutes but to recognise that things are not going well earlier (at about 10 minutes) and address any problems (especially any reversible causes).

At about 10 minutes

If the heart rate remains undetectable after 10 minutes of resuscitation, the team should consider effectiveness of ongoing resuscitation, reversible factors, the overall clinical picture and the views of the clinical team about continuing resuscitation.[378] Key clinical factors include specific circumstances known prior to delivery, the gestation of the baby, any wishes expressed by the family and the availability therapeutic hypothermia. It may also be appropriate at this stage, if staffing and circumstances allow, to update the parents of the lack of response despite resuscitative efforts.

By 20 minutes

The ILCOR and RCUK recommendation is that if, despite provision of all the recommended steps of resuscitation and exclusion of reversible causes, a newborn baby requires ongoing cardiopulmonary resuscitation for a prolonged period, it would be appropriate to discontinue resuscitation. A reasonable time frame to consider this is at 20 minutes or so after birth.[18]

The evidence for this recommendation comes from a meta-analysis of 13 studies in which researchers reported neurodevelopmental outcomes newborn infants who had an Apgar score of 0 (i.e. no heart rate) at ten minutes. Those 13 studies reported outcomes of 277 babies; 69% of whom had died by the time of follow-up.[379] 18% survived with moderate or severe impairment, 11% survived without any moderate or severe impairment and 2% were lost to follow up. The review also concluded that any specified duration of resuscitation was unlikely to uniformly predict survival or survival without impairment. It suggested that in any single case, relevant contextual factors include gestational age, the presence of congenital anomalies, the timing of perinatal insult, the perceived adequacy of resuscitative interventions performed, the family's stated preferences and values, and the availability of post-resuscitation resources such as neonatal intensive care and neuroprotective strategies must be considered as part of the decision-making process.

Withholding resuscitation

There are also situations where a more pertinent question might be 'should resuscitation be initiated?'. This might occur, for example, in the extremely preterm baby at 22 weeks gestation[144] or following the diagnosis of a life-limiting condition where the parents have opted not to terminate the pregnancy and the baby is to be offered palliative care.[380,381] The terminology used in such cases also needs to be considered and in the latter group, the term 'lethal' is best avoided because some babies with these malformations or underlying conditions can survive beyond the immediate newborn period.[382] It is important that the obstetric, midwifery and neonatal teams develop a consistent approach to these cases that takes into account the regional organisation of perinatal care and, above all, the views of the parents.[44]

Signs of life in even the most premature baby may persist for several hours after birth.[383] It is dishonest and hurtful to brush aside such signs of life and classify the baby as stillborn, especially when the family has witnessed these signs.

Most parents value having the opportunity to see and hold their dead or dying baby. Parents can readily understand that their baby is in the process of dying and can be grateful for the chance to share in this if reassured that the agonal gasps are not a sign of conscious pain or distress. They will want to be confident that the baby was assessed and that any chance of survival was not dismissed out of hand.

It can be a comfort to emphasise that a parent's love, care, comfort and warmth were the most important contributions to their baby's short life. To handle this situation with sensitivity and skill calls for experience. Therefore, junior members of staff should not be left to face such situations without support. It is important to manage pain and distress in a variety of non-pharmacological and pharmacological ways that prevent unnecessary separation of the parents and baby.[384]

Each department should agree a guideline for planning and managing births at extremely low gestational ages. You should familiarise yourself with your local guidelines but if you are in doubt about whether to intervene you should start resuscitation and get a senior colleague to come and assist you immediately.[385]

Definitions of live birth and stillbirth

Defining whether a baby is still born or born alive is extremely important to parents. It is also important from an epidemiological perspective, for example comparing stillbirth or neonatal death rates across different regions.

The UK and WHO definitions of stillbirth and live birth are shown in Tables 12.1 and 12.2. The WHO definitions are slightly more informative. It is important for families that when a baby dies, the classification of its death is made correctly. Incorrect classification, or disagreement (such as that between obstetricians and paediatricians about the presence or absence of signs of life) can cause distress and suffering for newly bereaved parents.

Pragmatic guidance for determining how to detect signs of life following spontaneous births before 24 weeks of gestation where, following discussion with parents, active survival-focused care is not appropriate has been produced (see https://timms.le.ac.uk/signs-of-life/).

Table 12.1   The legal definitions for live births and stillbirths in the UK

UK legal definitions	
Live birth	The legal definition of a live birth in the UK is 'a child born alive'.
Stillbirth	'A child which has issued forth from its mother after the 24th week of pregnancy and which did not at any time after being completely expelled from its mother breathe or show any other signs of life.'

Note: No gestational age is mentioned in the definition of livebirth however only babies born dead after 24 completed weeks of gestation are registered as stillbirths.

Table 12.2   The legal definitions for live births and stillbirths (fetal death) according to World Health Organisation (WHO)

WHO definitions	
Live birth	'The complete expulsion or extraction from its mother of a product of conception, irrespective of the duration of the pregnancy, which, after such separation, breathes or shows any other evidence of life, such as beating of the heart, pulsation of the umbilical cord, or definite movement of voluntary muscles, whether or not the umbilical cord has been cut or the placenta is attached; each product of such a birth is considered liveborn. Twins both born alive count as two live births but a child who dies from asphyxia caused by shoulder dystocia after delivery of the head but before delivery of the body is not a live birth.'
Stillbirth	'Death prior to complete expulsion or extraction from its mother of a product of conception, irrespective of the duration of pregnancy; the death is indicated by the fact that after such separation the fetus does not breathe or show any other evidence of life, such as beating of the heart, pulsation of the umbilical cord, or definite movement of voluntary muscles.'

12: Summary learning

When babies fail to respond to the standard NLS approach:

- Call for senior help
- Increase the inspired oxygen
- Secure the airway using a laryngeal mask or by intubating the baby
- Consider tracheal obstruction if there is inadequate chest movement despite the above
- If all the above fails, consider higher inflation pressures and/or longer inflation times.

Then:

- If bradycardia persists in the presence of adequate ventilation as judged by good chest movement for 30 s, then start chest compressions.
- If the baby remains bradycardic administer adrenaline, glucose and bicarbonate via a UVC (or intraosseous needle).
- Consider congenital abnormalities and exclude, or treat, reversible causes such as pneumothorax or blood loss.
- If the heart rate is still undetectable at 10 minutes prognosis is generally poor but some babies can survive. You should ensure that you have called for senior help. Do not stop resuscitation at this stage. Look for reasons why resuscitation might not be effective by going over A, B, C, D again.
- The decision to stop should only be taken after reviewing and addressing, where necessary, clinical factors and the effectiveness of resuscitation. A suggested timeframe for this is around 20 minutes.

My key take-home messages from this chapter are:

Human factors

The learning outcomes will enable you to:

Understand how to use a structured communication tool to improve sharing information

Gain insight into human factors which may be important in delivering effective care

Understand the importance of debriefing after a critical event

Introduction

Resuscitation of a newborn baby is often a very stressful situation, especially if it is unexpected or prolonged. Effective teamwork becomes increasingly important and complicated in prolonged or complicated resuscitations. In this chapter we discuss key elements which may be critical in the effective management of a resuscitation situation and how they can improve the likelihood of a successful outcome.

Communication

Those involved with any resuscitation event need to be able communicate effectively within and between teams. SBAR (Chapter 5) is a communication tool that has been developed to provide a structure to exchange information in a critical situation.

It has a number of potential advantages as it:

- provides a common platform across all healthcare disciplines
- ensures clarity when dealing with clinical situations
- streamlines communication and saves time.

The SBAR tool ensures that whoever is being spoken to has a clear idea of the problem, what the findings are, what is being done, and what is needed next.

It is vital that there is mutual respect within a team and that all involved with resuscitation feel able to communicate with each other. Just because someone is a junior member of the team, does not mean that their contribution is invalid; they may have spotted something very important and must feel empowered to point this out.[386-388] Communication with families is discussed in Chapters 6, 11 and 12.

Human factors

A widely used definition of clinical human factors is:

'Enhancing clinical performance through an understanding of the effects of teamwork, tasks, equipment, workspace, culture and organisation on human behaviour and abilities and application of that knowledge in clinical settings.'[389]

Practically these elements can be described in 4 main categories.

- Systems
- Processes
- Procedures
- Team working, human behaviour and abilities.

Systems

All healthcare systems are the product of a complex adaptive system of people, equipment, processes, and institutions working together.[390] Prior knowledge of the system in which you are delivering care will help with effective care planning, particularly in an emergency situation.

Different units will have different systems to prepare for babies needing resuscitation or stabilisation. For example, identifying high risk births requiring medical attendance, using a standard protocol for summoning the correct emergency team, advertising fixed locations for crash trolleys, standardising the equipment stored on the resuscitaire and the layout of the delivery room or theatre. Being familiar with these and many other factors help ensure the smooth running of a situation (see Chapter 6). Conversely, if the systems in place are inadequate, failure to deliver effective care is more likely as the margins for error are reduced.

An isolated system failure may not cause a problem but a combination can combine to create a life-threatening crisis.[372,291,392] For example, an initial failure to recognise a high-risk pregnancy, leading to the delivery of a baby requiring support without the neonatal team being present should not lead to a major life-threatening crisis as those in attendance should be able to begin stabilisation and resuscitation whilst calling for help. However, if there are multiple additional small system failures the situation can be quite different:

- The attendance of the neonatal team was delayed because of a failure to trigger an emergency call and the routine bleep system used instead.

- The neonatal team were further delayed arriving because several members of that team had just rotated to that hospital and are unfamiliar with the hospital layout. They had not been told exactly where to go when they were contacted.

- On arrival the neonatal team could not start to address the baby because the equipment in the room had not been checked following a previous delivery.

- There is a further delay in the arrival of the emergency trolley because an inexperienced member of staff does not know where to find it.

Thus, a combination of system failures leads to potentially significant delays in initiating newborn life support to the baby. This may in turn have important implications for their ongoing clinical trajectory.

Processes

The NLS algorithm is a good example of a standardised process which ensures that all involved are aware of the sequence of events. Individuals can anticipate needs, recognise omissions and be in a position to support.

Procedures

Whilst knowledge of the sequence is vital (process), equally important are the practical skills (procedures). Management of many clinical situations require interventions or procedures, such as mask inflation, suction, umbilical line insertion. These practical procedures need the right person to be in the right place, at the right time, with the right equipment and the right support team.

Team working, human behaviour and abilities

There are a number of 'non-technical' skills that enable effective team working. It is increasingly clear that the way we work together is crucial to the delivery of effective care, and can significantly affect the outcome of resuscitation.[393,394]

These non-technical skills include:

Situational awareness
Leadership and active followership
Decision-making
Communication skills
Task management
Management of errors

Situational awareness

This describes an awareness of what is going on around you. It requires an ability to rapidly sift information and focus on what is important whilst maintaining a global overview of a situation.

In newborn resuscitation those dealing with the baby are frequently concentrating on the airway and may focus solely on this potentially to the exclusion of other important factors, this is called fixation.[372,391,392] Fixation is the opposite of situational awareness. In a complex situation, with a clear leader who retains situational awareness, it can be safe for one person to be temporarily task fixated, for example, securing an airway by inserting a tracheal tube, as long as the team leader retains the global overview.

This overview, sometimes called the 'helicopter view', can be helpful to be able to consider the bigger picture and to coordinate more effectively, delegate tasks appropriately, monitor progress and identify any issues which may not have been dealt with.

Whilst there is some evidence that situational awareness tends to correlate with expertise, this does not mean that the individual detects all important events. In one simple experiment, volunteers who were adult resuscitators were shown videos of a simulated cardiac arrest that included a series of change-events designed to elicit perceptual errors; approximately 80% of inexperienced and 60% of experienced resuscitators missed the fact that the patient's oxygen supply had become disconnected.[395]

Teamworking, leadership and active followership

The team leader

Teams need to be organised with a clear leader. Ideally, the accepted team leader should be less 'hands on' during the resuscitation and more concerned with an oversight of the situation, but this is not always possible. The role of team leader is dynamic and depends on the skill mix and number in the team. The role may be handed over to the more senior clinicians as and when they arrive. Whilst a leader may not necessarily be the most senior member of the team, it is important that the leader is clearly identified and that the whole team are aware of any change in leadership.

Leadership can be defined in terms of the attributes of a leader or the process of leadership (Table 13.1). Clearer leadership is associated with more efficient cooperation in the team and also with better task performance and completion.

Table 13.1 Attributes of a team leader

The team leader needs to be able to:
Prioritise tasks
Allocate resources and delegate roles clearly
Call for additional help if needed
Moderate and control dialogue
Listen to those around whose input and observations may be invaluable
Reassess regularly and rectify problems
Deal with any conflict
Maintain a strategic overview of everything and plan ahead
Communicate effectively throughout the event

Good team leaders need communication, decision-making, organisational and delegating skills. They need to have the knowledge to be able to manage the situation effectively, to be able to recognise if things are going as planned and importantly if they are not, and when extra help is required.[396]

Active followership

Within a functioning team, being an active follower is just as important as having an effective leader. Attributes of an active team member/follower are shown in Table 13.2.

Table 13.2 Attributes of an active team member/follower

The active team member/follower needs to be able to:
Communicate clearly the clinical findings and actions they have taken to treat a patient
Be prepared to raise concerns about clinical or safety issues
Endeavour to help the team leader by listening carefully to briefing and instructions and communicating as necessary
Support and show respect for other team members and show tolerance towards hesitancy or nervousness in the emergency setting
Perform skills to the best of their ability
Admit when they cannot do something and need help
Be assertive enough to encourage debate about management if required or draw attention to a problem, but without being destructive
Feel sufficiently empowered to speak out and speak up in presence of errors

In some cases, staff may be called to a resuscitation and may not know one another, or what skills, background and experience they have. This can make it much more difficult for a potential team leader to give commands and to influence people to follow decisions and work together safely and efficiently. This difficulty can be minimised by a team briefing prior to the resuscitation if time allows.

All members of the resuscitation team are working towards a united common goal, which is to achieve the best possible outcome for the baby. By being a supportive team member, and actively following the leadership of the group, the team can work more functionally towards the common goal.

Knowing your team

Prior knowledge of the people you are working with, in terms of their experience and capabilities, can be very helpful, especially when delegating tasks and entrusting responsibility within a resuscitation scenario, as individuals within any group are heterogeneous in their abilities. This prior knowledge is not always possible given the composition of most resuscitation teams is multidisciplinary, and it should not be relied upon for an effective resuscitation.

Figure 13.1 The conscious competence learning model

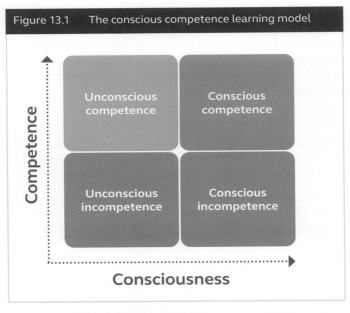

The conscious competence learning model (Figure 13.1) considers awareness of confidence and competence. There are 4 potential stages that learners may pass through when learning a new skill. Not all learners go through every stage and the NLS course aims to improve competence and with that bring appropriate confidence.

- Unconfident and incompetent
- Confident and incompetent
- Unconfident and competent
- Confident and competent

Do you know where you sit in this model?

What about other members of the team?

Confidence vs. competence

In addition to ability (competence) there is self-perception of ability (confidence) (Figure 13.1). They are not always concordant.

Those who are in the 'incompetent' stage need extra supervision. Those who are not confident, but are competent can manage, but need to be supported. Those who are confident but lack the competence may pose a potential risk and those who are confident and competent can be relied upon to perform. The aim of NLS and many similar training courses is to improve the competencies that underpin successful resuscitation, (and with increased competency, confidence).

Table 13.3 Levels of conflict that may occur during teamwork

1. Discussion	Where a team member may communicate awareness of a procedure, an item of kit, a protocol or an available expert and this may result in discussion. Discussion can be helpful in that it permits examination of a problem and should be encouraged irrespective of role, seniority or experience. The team leader should then acknowledge the information, then assess it and maybe use it to accomplish the treatment goal.
2. Disagreement	There may be disagreement over management. In this case the team leader should acknowledge the difference in opinion but must then be decisive after quickly exploring the alternative so as to minimise any delays.
3. Dispute	Dispute is perhaps the most difficult situation in an already stressful situation. Again, the team leader should acknowledge the difference of opinion, but then they need to assert their view and take action. If a team has a common goal (i.e. resuscitation of the baby) then conflict can usually be overcome by stressing the commitment to the common goal.

Decision-making

It is important that clear decisions are made, communicated and carried out in a timely manner, particularly in complex or prolonged resuscitations. The team leader should be a good communicator, a good listener and be decisive. The team leader should also be able to manage conflict which involves any team member proposing or suggesting something different to that already communicated. Whilst such conflict may raise issues that are important, it can also raise tension, cause delay in decision-making and damage the focus of the team or the team leader.

Often, these negative effects of conflict can be circumvented by stating the extreme urgency of the situation and the need to work as a team, emphasizing that the performance of every team member contributes to the overall success of the resuscitation. It may be helpful to state that the dispute (or the attitude of the disputing person) is not helping. In an extreme situation where the dispute threatens to impede the process, the team leader may ask someone to 'step out'. Three levels of conflict have been described (Table 13.3).[397]

Communication skills

Effective communication within a team is vital in any critical event. All dialogue needs to be precise. There is a natural tendency to use jargon during professional dialogue, including widespread use of abbreviations. Whilst in many cases this is helpful in rapidly communicating complex issues, it is important to ensure that what has been said has also been understood.

Do not assume everyone interprets things the same way.[398] This is especially true when considering abbreviations, which can mean very different things to different professions. For example, 'SGA' to a neonatologist means 'small for gestational age' but SGA to an anaesthetist has the completely different meaning of 'supraglottic airway'.

Above all, if the team is to work together effectively, communication should remain professional and avoid rudeness.[399]

Use closed loop communication

Instructions should be clearly stated to a named, specific individual who should respond to indicate they have heard and understood. This closes the communication loop.

For example, the person who is managing the airway may say to their colleague "I am going to give five inflation breaths. Dr Smith, could you please listen to the heart rate and tell me what it is after the fifth breath".

Dr Smith closes the communication loop by replying "I will reassess the heart rate after the fifth breath".[400]

Task management and role allocation

During any resuscitation there may be many tasks which need to be carried out, sometimes simultaneously. If the team is used effectively, it is possible to optimise management by dealing with more than one issue/problem at a time, accelerating the process and reaching a point of stability and definitive treatment earlier (Figure 13.2).

Effective delegation and task completion is integral to this.

An example of this is the management of a preterm baby at delivery, a scenario which undoubtedly benefits from prior planning to ensure a coordinated approach. A pre-brief can be extremely helpful in this scenario and many centres routinely use these for deliveries where additional support is anticipated. The sort of issues that can be anticipated in advance and roles allocated accordingly are as follows;

- Is the baby to be delivered on to the mother's abdomen to allow skin-to-skin and delayed cord clamping?
- Who will apply the plastic bag and hat?
- Who will assess the baby?
- If the baby requires resuscitation rather than stabilisation, will cord milking (if > 28 weeks) offer an alternative? If so, how will this be achieved?
- Who will clamp the cord and transfer to the resuscitaire?
- Who will place the saturation probe on the right wrist?
- Who will manage the airway?
- Is the resuscitaire set up correctly and appropriate sizes of face mask and other equipment available?
- Who will note the time/start the clock/take notes?
- Who will brief/support the parents?

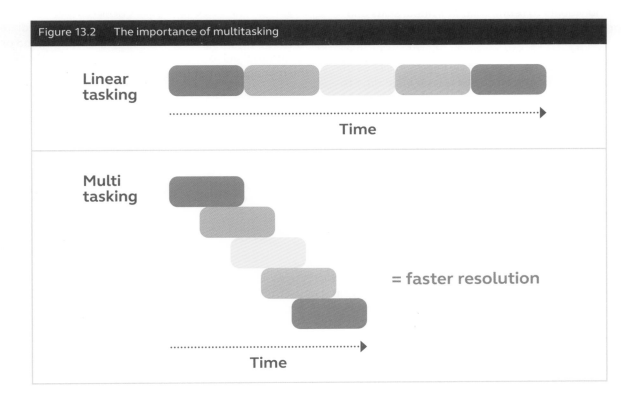

Figure 13.2   The importance of multitasking

Linear tasking

Time

Multi tasking

= faster resolution

Time

Errors

Mistakes do occur, and can take many forms.[401] Whilst some mistakes are minor and others are potentially catastrophic, it is the responsibility of everyone involved in dealing with a critical situation to identify any potential errors and communicate via the team leader to enable these to be dealt with effectively. Errors arise as a result of many factors (Table 13.4).

Table 13.4	Factors which might lead to error
Ignorance	Not everyone involved may know exactly how to deal with the situation
Assumption	Ensure that tasks have been completed rather than assuming that they have
Misinterpretation	Drawing incorrect conclusions from the information available
Fixation	Focusing exclusively on one aspect of care to the exclusion of other important areas
Arrogance	Greater self-belief than ability

Rehearsal

Rehearsal of situations in advance is a key factor in making systems, teams and individuals as efficient and effective as possible.[402] The NLS course was developed to introduce a structured, evidence-based approach to newborn life support. It provides an opportunity to begin to acquire the skills required to apply the algorithm effectively to a variety of situations, and to rehearse resuscitation skills. It enables individuals to refine their individual skills and their approach within a team.

Practicing in advance allows teams to identify potential problems before they happen, increasing the chances of a successful outcome. The NLS course is an ideal time to make mistakes, to practice a new approach and observe how others deal with difficult situations so that once back in the clinical area performance and outcomes are improved.

The NLS course teaches good practice, but adult learning and simulation literature show skills degradation occurs over time. It is the responsibility of an NLS provider to continue to practice the skills and team working taught on the course in their own clinical environments.[403] For those in busy units this will involve regular application of the skills in real life. Those in less busy or low-risk environments (for example, stand-alone midwife led units or community settings) will have to ensure they engage in regular manikin simulation sessions in order to maintain proficiency. If the skills learned are not practiced regularly, the provider will de-skill even if they have previously achieved the standard required to pass the course.

Debrief

Following any resuscitation, whether simulated or real, team members should have the opportunity to reflect on the event and discuss any safety issues.[404] These are sometimes referred to as 'hot debriefs'. Ideally, such debriefs need to involve all team members and take place as soon after the event as possible, before the shift changes and the ease of gathering the personnel involved is hindered. The identification of potential problems improves governance and ensures matters are dealt with in a timely and appropriate manner. Debriefs need to be non-judgmental, but constructive in how issues are dealt with.

There is increasing recognition of the additional value that is gained from providing 'psychological first aid' support after critical events, including newborn resuscitation. It aims to provide a compassionate and supportive presence for staff and to acknowledge the trauma associated with the event. By providing a safe space for staff to share their feelings, it can mitigate acute distress and promote processing of the event itself. Those facilitating such sessions should be appropriately trained to deliver this form of support, which differs considerably from the traditional medically-focused 'hot debrief'. In addition, they must have knowledge of the services or pathways available locally to enable them to signpost staff who are in need of additional or ongoing support.[402]

Where someone is facilitating a learning debrief following a simulation practice, they should ideally have been in a purely observational role whilst the simulation was ongoing. Those debriefing should have experience and training in how to undertake this. Through immediate debrief it may be possible to identify areas of good or suboptimal performance, which can then feed back into the management of future resuscitations.

13: Summary learning

SBAR is a useful tool to aid clarity of handover between professionals during critical events.

Managing a critical event such as newborn resuscitation effectively requires robust systems, clear processes, and competency with practical procedures.

Human factors can influence team performances both positively and negatively. Leadership and active followership are integral to effective functioning teams and promoting successful outcomes.

Rehearsal of, and debrief following, resuscitation situations enhance learning, support staff wellbeing and improve future management.

My key take-home messages from this chapter are:

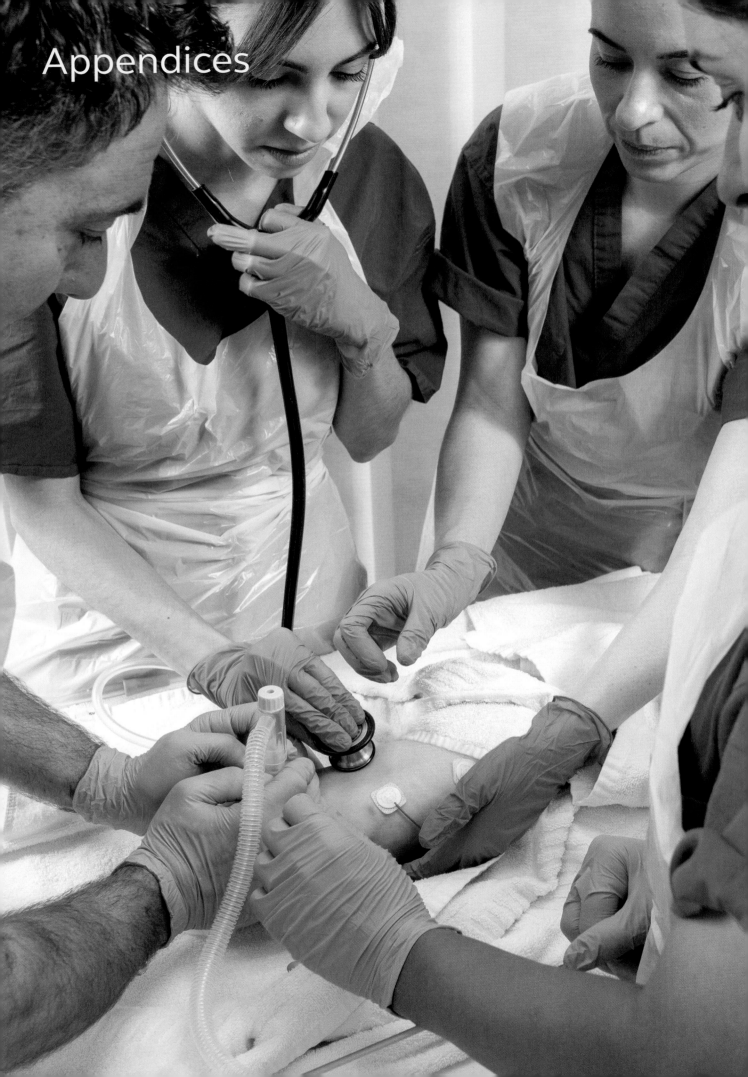

Appendices

Introduction and a cautionary note

Many things in this manual are consensus statements and one should always be sceptical of these. Just because everyone agrees you should do something a particular way does not mean that that really is the best way to do it. We would do well to remember the words of Sir Thomas Clifford Allbutt (1836–1925), English physician and inventor of the clinical thermometer:

"our path is cumbered with guesses, presumptions and conjectures, the untimely and sterile fruitage of minds which cannot wait for the facts and are ready to forget that the use of hypothesis lies not in the display of ingenuity but in the labour of verification".[405]

There are many controversies in the field of neonatal resuscitation and little strong experimental evidence is currently available to resolve them. Publication of an opinion, even in a highly reputable journal, does not mean that that opinion is correct. In 1951, a leading article was published in the Lancet entitled 'Anoxia in the Newborn' and confidently stated that "any method of attempting pulmonary expansion by blowing gases into the trachea under pressure must be condemned".[406] We now know that this is not only safe, but in many instances, it is a highly desirable practice. Similar 'own goals' include the common use of respiratory stimulants in the 1960s but we now know them to be both ineffective and potentially dangerous.[51]

Even as late as the 21st century, experts strongly recommended that the nose and mouth of the baby should be aspirated before the shoulders were delivered in labours complicated by meconium-stained liquor.[407] In 2004 this was shown in a large multi-centre randomised controlled study to be ineffective in preventing meconium aspiration syndrome.[211] We have also learnt that routine suctioning of the airway of any baby born through meconium-stained liquor is not only ineffective, but also potentially injurious, especially to those screaming babies whose airways were clearly patent.[212,408-411] More recently, we have learnt from randomised trials that routinely suctioning the trachea of even the floppiest of these babies does not prevent meconium aspiration syndrome, and that spending time removing meconium may delay the onset of basic resuscitation.[208-210,411]

Many other examples of ineffective treatments exist. Future work will hopefully resolve some of these controversies, but others will certainly arise to take their place.

Much of the physiological evidence on which the strategies of neonatal resuscitation are based relates to sudden total anoxia. In real-life intermittent, partial hypoxia of varying severity, frequency and duration, with or without accompanying ischaemia, is the more common pattern of intrapartum insult affecting the fetus. The physiological response to this pattern of stresses is less well explored and may be subtly different. Furthermore, the response of a chronically stressed baby whose intrauterine growth has been compromised may well be different to that of a well grown baby facing significant problems for the first time. Heart rate responses to stress in labour differ between male and female babies. It is also likely that the quality and nature of any fetal responses will vary with varying degrees of fetal maturity.

While the current enthusiasm for detailed protocols continues it should be remembered that a protocol is only as good as the experimental evidence on which it is based. The advice in this manual constitutes a guide to resuscitation at birth. It represents the collective opinion of many with extensive personal experience of performing neonatal resuscitation as well as teaching the subject. Increasingly structured systematic reviews help inform practice, but these can only analyse evidence that is available. The advice given does not define the only way that resuscitation at birth should be performed. We merely suggest that it is an accepted view of how resuscitation at birth can be carried out both safely and effectively.

Controversies

There are several controversial areas in newborn resuscitation. Most are capable of generating an amount of intense argument quite out of proportion to their importance. Nevertheless, these controversies still cause distress, confusion and debate. This section will attempt to set out some of the evidence on either side of the various debates and put the arguments in context.

Use of CPAP and/or PEEP at birth in the term or near-term baby

When attending the delivery of preterm infants, one is more commonly involved in stabilisation ('assisted transition') of a fragile infant rather than resuscitation of a nearly dead one. Gentle support of spontaneous respiration using CPAP, rather than immediate intubation, is now widely recognised as the optimum mode of respiratory support in most preterm babies.

Three large, randomised trials have examined the strategy of initial stabilisation on nasal CPAP versus, what was then, the conventional management of intubation and surfactant administration in preterm babies; the CPAP Or INtubation at birth (COIN) trial,[215] the Surfactant Positive Pressure and Oxygen Randomized Trial (SUPPORT),[412] and the Vermont Oxford Network Delivery Room Management (VON DRM) trial.[413] These, and several smaller trials, were included in a Cochrane meta-analysis that concluded that, compared to mechanical ventilation, prophylactic nasal CPAP in very preterm infants reduces the incidence of chronic lung disease and the combined outcome of death or chronic lung disease.[414] There is, therefore, good evidence for the use of CPAP or PEEP in the preterm baby as it facilitates lung aeration and maintains lung volume.

The evidence for use of CPAP in term and near-term infants is less clear.[219,220] A number of retrospective cohort studies have suggested that delivery room CPAP in term and near-term infants may be associated with an increased incidence of pneumothorax or pulmonary air leak.[221-223] Why this might be so is unclear, but since the 2010 newborn resuscitation guidelines and CPAP (especially face mask CPAP) became increasingly available and was easy to use, the proportion of term infants receiving respiratory support increased substantially. Babies in whom a 'wait and see' approach would have previously been taken would be more likely to receive CPAP. In one study a quarter of low-risk babies born by caesarean section received some form of respiratory support.[415]

Chest compressions – when to switch from the newborn 3:1 to the paediatric 15:2 compression to ventilation ratio

Chest compressions used in resuscitation may be administered in a number of different ways, in a variety of ratios and may (or may not) be synchronised with ventilation breaths. Until recently, the ways in which chest compressions are delivered were poorly researched and evidence remains sparse.

A major difference between the newborn and paediatric guidelines is in the ratio of compressions to ventilations. The ILCOR evaluation of the evidence for these two groups arrived at different conclusions. Newborn babies and those on neonatal units, special care units and postnatal wards should usually receive 3 compressions to 1 ventilation (a 3:1 ratio) as the reason for resuscitation is most likely to be respiratory and this ratio is most likely to deliver an appropriate ventilation rate. If a baby is thought to have a primary cardiac cause for arrest, consideration should be given to using a ratio of 15 compressions to 2 ventilations (15:2 ratio).

A baby who has successfully adapted to extrauterine life and has subsequently collapsed and presented to the emergency department or collapsed on a joint neonatal/paediatric medical and surgical intensive care unit should be resuscitated according to paediatric life support algorithms with a 15:2 compression to ventilation ratio.

For pragmatic reasons it is suggested that the ratio of compressions to ventilations should be that with which most people are familiar; i.e. use 3:1 in a neonatal or maternity setting and 15:2 in a paediatric or emergency department.

Sodium bicarbonate

This manual recommends that drugs should only be used in those very rare situations where the heart rate has not responded to adequate lung aeration, ventilation and chest compressions. Adrenaline is probably the drug of first choice, particularly if administered intravascularly (or if this unavailable intraosseous route).
Tracheal administration is a less effective alternative. However scientific evidence to support the use of any drug in newborn resuscitation is lacking.

Many authorities have significant reservations about using bicarbonate.[297,416,417] On closer inspection, these reservations relate to the practice of routinely correcting acidosis following resuscitation or routinely giving an infusion of bicarbonate during resuscitation; reservations which are entirely reasonable.[418] However, it does not follow that bicarbonate should be disregarded altogether.

Good quality evidence for or against the use of sodium bicarbonate in human newborn babies who are severely compromised due to hypoxia is also lacking. Only one small (under-powered) randomised trial in human newborn babies requiring resuscitation has looked at the effects of sodium bicarbonate.

This study, reported in two separate publications.[419,420] In these babies who were still receiving positive pressure ventilation at 5 min randomisation was to receive sodium bicarbonate (n=27) or a dextrose placebo (n=28). The investigators concluded bicarbonate does not help to improve survival or immediate neurological outcome. There are some issues with the study; that only 12 of the group treated with bicarbonate (and 11 of the placebo group) received chest compressions throws an element of doubt into the validity of the study. This would not be in keeping with the standard NLS algorithm in that drugs are advocated only after chest compressions have been shown to be ineffective. There were also inequalities in the baseline characteristics in that more babies in the bicarbonate arm had lower mean Apgar scores at one and five minutes, more were born through meconium-stained liquor and more were given adrenaline.

Some early animal studies examined the effect of injecting either respiratory stimulants or base intravenously, in these studies the alkali used was the organic base, trometamol (formerly better known as tris-hydroxymethyl-aminomethane or THAM) rather than bicarbonate. All the animals (fetal monkeys) were known to have taken their last gasp and were in terminal apnoea.[52] Respiratory stimulants (lobeline or nikethamide) caused hypotension, whereas THAM (0.5% molar solution with 3.5% dextrose, with the pH adjusted to 8.85) improved both heart rate and blood pressure and the re-emergence of gasping sufficient to allow successful resuscitation using positive pressure ventilation.

This is why this text continues to recommend that sodium bicarbonate be considered in prolonged resuscitations provided adequate lung aeration, ventilation and chest compression do not achieve an increase in heart rate.

Unfortunately, the impact of administering base on the effectiveness of adrenaline had not been investigated in the experiment described above.[52] Animal data shows that the binding of adrenaline to its receptors in the myocardium is significantly impaired by lactic acidosis[421] and studies on lymphocyte beta-adrenergic receptors suggests the same is true in humans.[287] Whether this is also true of the more important alpha-adrenergic receptors is unknown.

Intratracheal adrenaline

Human infant data on which to base guidelines for adrenaline during neonatal resuscitation are also lacking. Even fewer data exist regarding which route might be best. In order to overcome some of the delay associated with intravenous administration of adrenaline at newborn resuscitation it has been suggested that adrenaline can be effective when given down the tracheal tube into the lungs.[272] Few of the animal studies of this technique have been done in newborn animals whose lungs have just been aerated.

The dose required to be effective when given by this route appears to be somewhat higher than the intravenous dose. In adult resuscitation it is effective provided a dose of at least 2 mg is given (i.e. twice that via the intravenous route).[422] However, adult lungs are different anatomically and physiologically and are usually fully aerated. In newborn piglets, standard doses given intravenously had measurable effects on carotid blood pressure, but the same doses given via the tracheal tube did not.[423]

One case series of intratracheal and intravenous adrenaline showed a response was more common after an intravenous adrenaline than after a similar dose of tracheal adrenaline.[226] This is consistent with evidence extrapolated from animal models indicating that higher doses (50–100 microgram kg^{-1}) of tracheal adrenaline may be required to achieve the increased blood adrenaline concentrations and haemodynamic responses seen after intravenous administration.[424,425]

The presence of fetal lung fluid has an impact on absorption from the trachea; in an ovine model of asphyxia serum adrenaline levels were lower in newborn lambs than those aged 1–3 days following tracheal administration of 100 micrograms kg^{-1} of adrenaline. The proportion of lambs showing return of spontaneous circulation was also higher in the 1–3 day old group.[426]

Although it has been widely assumed that adrenaline can be administered faster by the tracheal route than the intravenous route, no clinical trials have evaluated this hypothesis. Whether effective or not, if you want to give tracheal adrenaline then a tracheal tube needs to be in place.

Naloxone for the apnoeic baby and a history of maternal opiate abuse

Many guidelines on resuscitation at birth warn against giving naloxone to the baby of an opiate abusing mother for fear of inducing fits. As justification all quote the same single brief case report of fits in a newborn baby that was attributed to this cause.[427] In this report, seizures are reported to have started two minutes after the baby received a 200 microgram intramuscular dose of naloxone shortly after birth, and to have stopped thirty minutes later just as soon as a 100 microgram kg^{-1} bolus of morphine was given intravenously. There are, for many people, additional details that are missing from the report:

- the baby was delivered by caesarean section for 'fetal distress' although the nature of this is not given

- there were no umbilical cord gases stated

- the baby only received naloxone after failing to breathe spontaneously at four minutes of age (suggesting that the respiratory depression may have been caused by the very 'fetal distress' that led to the caesarean section in the first place).

This remains, after over thirty years, the only published report of such a complication and, since no other case has ever been reported to the UK or other licensing authorities. That said, the use of naloxone has declined substantially since the report was published and there has been a general move away from naloxone use as a 'drug of resuscitation' These changes, alone, might explain the absence of any further reports through any pharmacovigilance schemes such as the Medicines and Healthcare products Regulatory Agency's yellow card scheme.

There are, nonetheless, anecdotal reports of acute opiate withdrawal symptoms in babies whose mothers have been taking opiates and where the baby was given naloxone shortly after birth. The withdrawal symptoms involved agitation and jitteriness and started in the delivery room, however, none have been seizures. There is one report of naloxone causing unexpected abrupt cardiac arrest in a ventilated very preterm baby who had been given a 10-fold overdose of morphine.[428] The mechanism for the cardiac arrest is unclear but it is known that naloxone potentiates the release of adrenaline in hypoxic sheep[429] and augments the catecholamine surge at birth.[430]

Data regarding naloxone use is sparse and suggests little clinical benefit.[431,432] The priority must be to address A, B, C (and possibly D) before considering naloxone and then only in those babies known to have been exposed to maternal opiates during labour.

Intraosseous (IO) access

Recent data suggest that the IO route can be effective in the resuscitation of preterm and term infants in the intensive care unit when alternative venous access proves difficult or impossible to establish.[269] However, it is difficult to justify the insertion of such a device into the bone of a newborn baby when umbilical venous catheterisation so easily provides central venous access of known efficacy.

Whether there are advantages to the IO route is unclear. A recent meta-analysis in adults of intravenous and intraosseous routes reported sparse data but suggested that in observational studies the intravenous route was better, but in RCTs there was no advantage to using the intraosseous over the intravenous route.[433]

The most recent ILCOR guidance suggests

"umbilical venous catheterization as the primary method of vascular access during newborn infant resuscitation in the delivery room. If umbilical venous access is not feasible, the intraosseous route is a reasonable alternative for vascular access during newborn resuscitation".

Reasons for difficulty might include the rare abnormalities of the umbilical cord (e.g. exomphalos or gastroschisis).[434-436]

Maternity units may not have ready access to the equipment for intraosseous access and most staff, with the possible exception of paediatric medical staff, may not have been trained in this technique. Given the infrequency with which this technique might be used (and that the equipment required might not be readily available) it is suggested that all units where babies are born are trained how to access both the equipment and expertise to use the IO route as well as the intravenous route.

The other situation where it might be useful is in resuscitation outside labour ward (e.g. in the Emergency Department) where staff might be more familiar with the intraosseous route.[437]

'Sustained' inflations

The Newborn Life Support course has long advocated the use of what it calls 'inflation breaths' using the term to describe the 2–3 s aeration breaths given at the start of resuscitation. These have sometimes been called sustained in that they are longer than ventilation breaths. The inflation breaths described in this manual (and its predecessors) are not to be confused with 'sustained inflation' breaths used in several studies; all of these are breaths that are sustained for at least 10 s (in some cases up to 20 s).

Early work describing the first breaths of life in healthy term babies had shown the first breaths tend to be deeper and longer overall than subsequent breaths and are characterized by a short deep inspiration followed by a prolonged expiratory phase.[100,182,438,439] It is thought that babies breathe out against partially closed vocal cords which generates back pressure to the lungs and helps clear the lung fluid. This process is assisted by the diaphragm slowing expiration. This 'expiratory braking' facilitates the distribution of air within the lungs and assists in the formation of the functional residual capacity (FRC).[440]

An early study of resuscitation of compromised hypoxic babies showed that a similar increase in the tidal volume and the FRC could be achieved with sustained inflations.[138] The 2–3 s 'inflation breaths' of the NLS course were informed by these data.

Table A1	Duration and pressures used in the sustained lung inflation arms of RCTs included in the Cochrane meta-analysis[441]
Study	Sustained lung inflation duration and inspiratory pressure
Lindner et al (2005)[442]	Inspiratory pressure of 20 cm water for 15 s If response was not satisfactory: 2 further sustained inflation of 15 s duration at 25 and 30 cm water respectively
Lista et al (2015)[443]	Inspiratory pressure of 25 cm water for 15 s then PEEP of 5 cm water
Schwaberger et al (2015)[444]	Initial sustained inflation of 30 cm water sustained for 15 s Repeated if HR < 100 min^{-1}
Mercadante et al (2016)[445]	Inspiratory pressure of 25 cm water for 15 s then PEEP of 5 cm water Sustained inflation repeated if HR < 100 min^{-1}
Abd El-Fattah et al (2017)[446]	4 different arms: inspiratory pressure of either 15 or 20 cm water sustained for either 10 or 20 s
El-Chimi et al (2017)[447]	Initial sustained inflation of 20 cm water for 15 s, followed by PEEP of 5 cm water. Second and third sustained inflations given if needed: • 25 cm water for 15 s, followed by PEEP of 6 cm water • 30 cm water for 15 s, followed by PEEP of 7 cm water
Jiravisitkul et al (2017)[448]	Inspiratory pressure of 25 cm water for 15 s Option for repeat sustained inflation (same parameters) if HR 60–100 min^{-1} and/or poor respiratory effort
Ngan et al (2017)[449]	Two sustained inflations using pressure of 24 cm water. Duration of first breath was 20 s. Duration of second breath was 10 or 20 s depending on exhaled CO_2 value
Schmölzer et al (2018)[450]	Two sustained inflations of 20 s during chest compressions at a pressure of 24 cm water
Kirpalani et al (2019)[185]	Inspiratory pressure of 25 cm water for 15 s Option for repeat sustained inflation (same parameters) if HR 60–100 min^{-1} and/or poor respiratory effort

The most recent Cochrane meta-analysis[441] reviewed outcomes from ten trials of sustained lung inflation (> 1 seconds) versus standard inflation (≤ 1 s). The duration and pressures of the sustained lung inflations varied considerably across the trials (Table A1).

It can be seen from the table that across all the trials the shortest sustained breath was 15 seconds which is considerably longer that the inflation breaths advocated on the NLS course.

These trials were also included in a meta-analysis by the ILCOR Neonatal Life Support Task Force.[184] The definition of sustained inflation was slightly different in this review (> 5 s versus > 1 s in the Cochrane review) but because none of the trials looked at sustained breaths shorter than 15 s, the different definitions had no impact on the findings which were essentially similar in that neither were able to recommend the use of sustained inflations. Both were keen to highlight the outcomes from the SAIL study which was not only the biggest of the included studies, but which, importantly, was stopped early due to an excess of deaths in the sustained lung inflation arm in infants < 28 weeks.[185]

The NLS course will continue to use the term 'inflation breaths' for the 2–3 s duration breaths at the start of resuscitation but cannot recommend 'sustained inflations' of > 5 s duration unless this is within the context of a properly conducted clinical trial.

Can cord gases tell us when the hypoxic insult began?

If there are concerns that the baby has been significantly compromised it can be helpful to obtain blood for measurement of pH, base deficit and lactate from an umbilical artery and the vein (i.e. a 'paired' blood gas).[346-348,350]

Whilst the results of these do not usually impact on the resuscitation (sometimes the result is not known until after the resuscitation is finished), they can nonetheless provide some useful information about the gas exchange processes in the minutes leading up to delivery. The analyses must, however, be done in a timely fashion particularly as they may impact on post-resuscitation

care and the consideration of the use of therapeutic hypothermia.[350]

If paired arterial and venous samples are obtained it is the arterial sample that shows a marginally lower pH, higher carbon dioxide and lactate and a worse base excess (this is different from the usual situation where venous blood gases are worse). This is because the umbilical arterial gases reflect the status of the fetus, whereas the umbilical venous gases reflect the ability of the placenta to deal with the excess carbon dioxide and lactic acid from the fetus. The range of 'normal values' from 146 uncomplicated vaginal deliveries at term[451] is shown in Table A2.

In general, the lower range for normal arterial pH extends to at least 7.10 and that for venous pH to at least 7.20. There is no consensus as to what constitutes significant acidosis; the pH values that have been used to define acidosis range from 7.00 to 7.20.[452,453] There is a poor relationship between Apgar score, need for resuscitation and eventual neurodevelopmental outcome and cord pH; whilst only 2% of babies with a normal Apgar score have a pH < 7.10, most babies with a cord blood pH between 7.00 and 7.10 will have a normal Apgar score. It is only when the cord blood pH reaches levels less than 7.00 that low Apgar scores become common.[454]

In an acutely and continuously compromised fetus where placental gas exchange is impaired, there is a progressive fall in pH from 7.32 at 5 min and to 7.00 at 10 min.[455]

Once severe acidosis is present, the likelihood of adverse sequelae rises sharply with worsening acidosis. Historical data showed the numbers of infants with HIE increased steadily with worsening cord pH from 12% with cord pH < 7.0, 33% with cord pH < 6.9, 60% with cord pH < 6.8, and 80% with cord pH < 6.7.[455] No infants survived when the cord pH was < 6.6.[455]

When paired venous and arterial umbilical cord samples are taken it is possible to get some indication of the timing of the hypoxic insult in terms of it being 'acute' or 'chronic'. This is because the fetus produces carbon dioxide and lactic acid, both of which are removed by the placenta. Most cases of fetal acidosis during labour are acute in onset, and in most cases the placenta retains

Table A2 Normal ranges for blood gas parameters from umbilical arterial and venous samples from uncomplicated vaginal deliveries of term babies

	Arterial		Venous	
	Mean (± 1SD)	Range	Mean (± 1SD)	Range
pH	7.28 (± 0.05)	7.15–7.43	7.35 (± 0.05)	7.24–7.49
PCO_2 (kPa)	6.56 (± 1.12)	4.15–9.91	5.09 (± 0.75)	3.09–6.56
PO_2 (kPa)	2.40 (± 0.83)	0.51–4.51	3.89 (± 0.79)	2.05–6.42
Bicarbonate (mmol L⁻¹)	22.3 (± 2.5)	13.3–27.5	20.4 (± 2.1)	15.9–24.7

the ability to compensate for much of the excess acids produced by the hypoxic fetus. However, if the insult is profound and prolonged, then this compensatory mechanism is overwhelmed. Thus a 'bad' umbilical arterial gas paired with a 'better' venous gas is suggestive of a more recent event, whereas if both arterial and venous samples are bad then the event is more likely to have been more prolonged.[348]

Other factors, however, come into play and the cord blood gases should not be viewed in isolation. Differences between arterial and venous samples may be pronounced in nuchal cords (i.e. when the umbilical cord becomes wrapped at least once around the fetal neck)[456] and reduced when there is placental abruption.[457] If the insult was a cord obstruction that is released shortly before delivery, it is possible that the umbilical arterial and venous gases can be normal despite severe intrapartum compromise and even fetal demise.[458]

Umbilical cord gases can still be obtained after delayed cord clamping, however there are some suggestions that various parameters can change significantly during the period when the cord remains unclamped; Giovannini and colleagues compared immediate sampling from the unclamped cord with later sampling from the same cord after it had been clamped at 3 minutes. Babies were delivered either vaginally or by caesarean section and there had been no CTG evidence of fetal distress. They found that the samples after 3 minutes were more acidotic than those taken earlier; in babies delivered by caesarean section the worsening was a mixed respiratory and metabolic picture, whereas for vaginally delivered babies it was metabolic.[459] This would suggest that further research is required in relation to umbilical cord gases when undertaking DCC and that sampling after DCC may be an unreliable indicator of fetal wellbeing.

Umbilical cord gases provide some indication of the extent of compromise in many cases, however they cannot, in isolation, be used to determine the timing of the hypoxic insult. Additional information about the antenatal health of both the mother and the fetus, as well as information about events during labour must be taken into account.

Scoring systems

The Apgar score and Sarnat grading are common scoring systems used to classify babies at birth or soon after.

Modified Sarnat grading is used to grade encephalopathy, particularly if therapeutic hypothermia is being considered. Neither score should be recorded simply as a number. A detailed description of the baby is essential.

(a) The Apgar score

The Apgar score, calculated by assigning scores to various physiological parameters (Table A3), has major limitations. It was originally devised for use as 'a basis for discussion and comparison of the results of obstetric practices, types of maternal pain relief and the effects of resuscitation'.[460] It is of some use in retrospectively categorising groups of babies, but of no use in the clinical management of individual babies.[461] Virginia Apgar, who was an obstetric anaesthetist, did not expect the score to predict mortality in individual babies but she did hope it might reveal a relationship between condition at birth and long-term neurological outcome. [462]

A large cohort study from Norway showed that babies with a very low Apgar score (≤ 3 at 5 minutes) had a 11% risk of showing signs of cerebral palsy (if they survive to one year) as compared with a risk of 0.1% for babies with a very high score (nine or more).[463] However, this tells us little about the cause of the cerebral palsy. Babies with low scores could include those with a longstanding problem prior to birth, those who had suffered a recent adverse event before birth as well as those who suffered an insult during birth.

The study did show that almost 90% of survivors with a very low Apgar score do not have cerebral palsy and 80% of those with cerebral palsy had an Apgar score of seven or more. This correlates well with data from an American study which showed that 80% of survivors with a score of Apgar three or less were entirely normal at school age.[463]

Virginia Apgar certainly drew attention to features which are important in assessing condition at birth but assigning scores to these features seems to have been much less

Table A3 The Apgar score is calculated by assigning scores of 0–2 to five physiological and behavioural observations. Resulting in an overall score of 0–10

Score	0	1	2
Colour	Pale/blue	Body pink, extremities blue	Pink
Heart rate	Absent	Less than 100	More than 100
Response to stimulation	Nil	Some movement	Cry
Muscle tone	Limp	Some flexion of extremities	Well flexed
Respiratory effort	Absent	Weak cry or hypoventilation	Good

helpful. The respiratory and heart rate scores are more important than the other items and the total score on its own is particularly uninformative. Heart rate is only variable that has some association with outcome.

While it has long been assumed that a close relationship exists between the Apgar score and pH and umbilical blood gas status at birth, Sykes et al showed that this is not so.[464] Only 21% of babies with a one minute Apgar score < 7, and 19% of babies with a 5 minute score < 7 had an umbilical artery blood pH < 7.1. Conversely 73% with severe acidosis had a 1 minute ≥ 7, while 86% had a 5 minute score ≥ 7.

In practice, the Apgar score is usually recorded retrospectively and subjectively. For these reasons it may be highly unreliable. If you record the Apgar score, a written description of all the characteristics used to assign the score must also be recorded as well as the details of any resuscitation.

(b) Sarnat grading (modified Sarnat score)

In a baby who receives significant resuscitation at birth and who goes on to show signs of encephalopathy it is important to document the neurological state regularly over the first few days and not just at birth. The most useful system for this purpose is the modified Sarnat grading (Table A4).[465]

Early seizures (before 48 hours) are worrying, but signs of a moderate or severe encephalopathy at 24–48 hours correlate more closely with outcomes two years and eight years later.[466] A recorded modified Sarnat grade at 48 hours in a term baby suspected of intrapartum 'asphyxia' is prognostically more useful than the Apgar score at birth. Early neonatal seizures are not always due to intrapartum hypoxia; nor is early neonatal encephalopathy, but intrapartum hypoxia is certainly the commonest cause of early encephalopathy in the term baby. The likelihood that the encephalopathy is related to intrapartum events is enhanced if there is other evidence of organ dysfunction.

Table A4 The Modified Sarnat score for evaluating babies with suspected hypoxic-ischaemic brain injury based upon their neurologic features

Domain	Stage 1	Stage 2	Stage 3
Seizures	None	Common focal or multifocal seizures	Uncommon (excluding decerebration) or frequent seizures
Level of consciousness	Normal or hyper alert	Lethargic Decreased activity in an infant who is aroused and responsive Can be irritable to external stimuli	Stuperose/ comatose Not able to rouse and unresponsive to external stimuli
Spontaneous activity when awake or aroused	Active Vigorous does not stay in one position	Less than active Not vigorous	No activity whatsoever
Posture	Moving around and does not maintain only one position	Distal flexion, complete extension or frog – legged position	Decerebrate with or without stimulation (all extremities extended)
Tone	Normal – resists passive motion Hypertonic, jittery	Hypotonic or floppy, either focal or general	Completely flaccid like a 'rag doll'
Primitive reflexes:			
Suck	Vigorously sucks finger or ET tube	Weak suck	Completely absent
Moro	Normal extension of limbs followed by flexion	Incomplete	Completely absent
Autonomic system:			
Pupil	Normal size Reactive to light	Constricted (< 3mm) but react to light	Fixed dilated, skew gaze not reactive to light
Heart rate	Normal > 100 min⁻¹	Bradycardia (< 100 min⁻¹ variable up to 120 min⁻¹)	Heart rate: variable inconsistent rate, irregular, may be bradycardic
Respirations	Normal	Periodic irregular breathing effort	Completely apnoeic requiring positive pressure ventilation

The threshold for recognising mild (Sarnat Grade 1) encephalopathy probably varies in different centres, but most units can expect to encounter 2–3 babies with Grade 2 or Grade 3 encephalopathy per 1000 livebirths. Signs of encephalopathy need to be documented daily; better documentation of the duration of symptoms is likely to improve the prognostic power of the Sarnat grading system.

Personal Protective Equipment (PPE) in newborn resuscitation

The SARS-CoV-2 pandemic brought into focus considerable thought about appropriate levels of PPE needed during all resuscitation situations in all age groups. Two other coronavirus infections – severe acute respiratory syndrome associated coronavirus (SARS-CoV) in 2002 and the Middle East respiratory syndrome coronavirus (MERS-CoV) in 2012 – also affected pregnant individuals but caused more severe disease.[467] Nonetheless many lessons were learnt from those infections that informed the use of PPE during the SARS-CoV-2 pandemic that began in 2019.

Resuscitation of the newborn is unique in that it usually results in caring for two (or more) patients; both of whom can pose different levels of risk. The risks of transmission of SARS-CoV-2 to the attending resuscitators from mother and baby can be reduced through appropriate use of PPE.

The need for PPE, however, is not limited to SARS-CoV-2 infections as other pathogens can be transmitted in bodily secretions or blood. The concepts about assessing risk, choosing appropriate PPE and being able to deliver planned resuscitation measures whilst wearing that PPE are generalizable.

Risk assessment

In assessing the risk of transmission of a pathogen to members of the resuscitation team, the following factors need to be considered:

- Is there a known (confirmed or suspected) potentially transmissible pathogen in either mother or baby?

- What are the main modes of transmission of that pathogen e.g. contaminated body fluids, droplet or aerosol spread?
- What is known about the transmissibility of the pathogen?
- Are there known groups of individuals that are more vulnerable to catching or becoming unwell with this pathogen? Are they part of the resuscitation team?
- What level of PPE is needed?
- Who poses the greatest risk to the resuscitation team; the mother, the baby or both?
- Can exposure be limited by minimising the number in the resuscitation team? And who should be in that team?
- Where will newborn life support be carried out? Does resuscitation in a separate room provide greater protection against transmission?[468]
- Does resuscitation equipment needed to be modified e.g. the use of HEPA filters in T-pieces or self-inflating bags?
- Are there alternatives to standard equipment that can offer more protection e.g. videolaryngoscopy versus standard laryngoscopy?
- If post-resuscitation care is needed where will this occur, how will the baby be transferred and what isolation or barrier nursing measures are required?

Levels of PPE

Levels of PPE describe increasing amounts of protection and help explain what may be needed in different situations. A primary consideration in determining the level of PPE is whether aerosol generating procedures are necessary for patient care. The characteristics of droplet versus airborne transmission are shown in Table A5.

Exact definitions of levels of PPE may vary (and may change with time) but one example is:

Table A5   Droplet versus airborne transmission and how this impacts on the PPE requirements.[469]

	Droplet transmission	Airborne transmission
Particle size	More than 5 micrometres	5 micrometres or smaller
Distance of travel from source	3–6 feet (1–2 metres)	Can exceed 6 feet (2 metres)
Route of infection	Mucus membranes of the nose, mouth and eyes	As for droplets but also inhalation to lower respiratory tract
Type of PPE required*	**Level 1** Includes a fluid resistant surgical face mask (FSRM)	**Level 2** Includes an FFP3 face mask or N95 respirator mask
*Follow relevant local, regional or national guidelines		

Level 1 PPE

- Single pair of gloves
- Disposable plastic apron
- Fluid-resistant surgical face mask
- Eye protection if you feel there is a risk of patient coughing, or splash or droplet exposure.

Level 2 PPE

- Single pair of gloves
- Long sleeved fluid-resistant gown
- FFP3 face mask or N95 respirator face mask
- Eye protection (visor which can be disposable or reusable).

FFP3 (or equivalent N95 masks) do not fit everybody equally well and face mask fit testing is advised prior to their adoption for use in situations with a risk of aerosol transmission.

Where face mask fit testing should be done in a planned and timely way before being exposed to resuscitation situations with a risk of infection transmission. A change in the supply (e.g. due to a supply from a different manufacturer) should prompt a repeat of the face mask

Figure A1 The team stabilising a baby born to a mother who had tested positive for SARS-CoV-2 showing the amount of PPE that was required to protect them from infection. The team are stabilising the baby in a room outside the obstetric theatre.

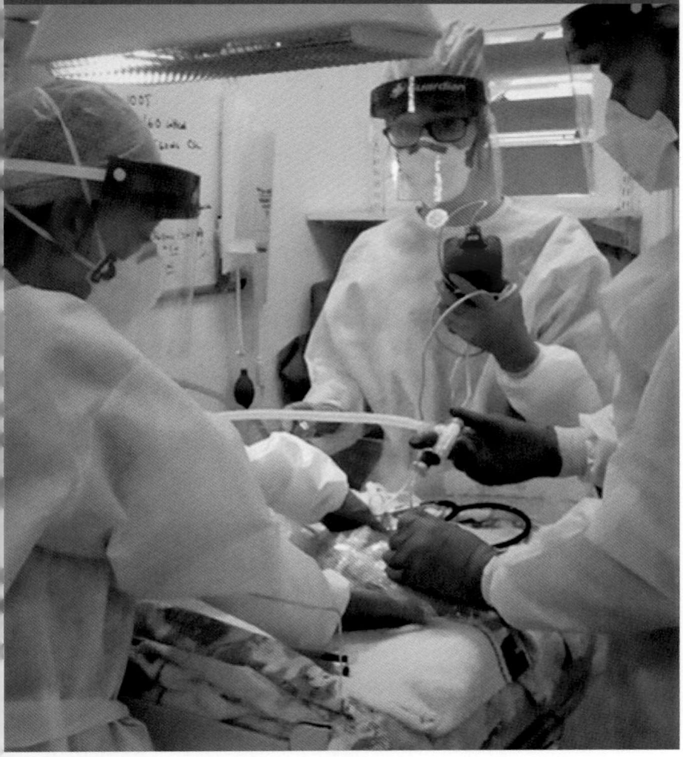

fit testing as not all masks are identical. Similarly, due to differences in facial structure, no single mask is suitable for all people. Availability of PPE needs to be considered when planning resuscitation services.

Impact of PPE on teamworking and communication

PPE can disrupt interpersonal communication in teams (Figure A1). Face coverings can obscure both verbal and non-verbal communication; they decrease speech intelligibility particularly in a noisy resuscitation environment.[470] In addition, speech can be further distorted through devices (e.g. speaker phones) used to communicate with team members on standby outside of the resuscitation room. In simulations, these difficulties are reported to cause problems such as poorly synchronised chest compressions, incomplete resuscitation records, and delays in contacting addition personnel. There is also reduced shared situational awareness and team coordination.[471]

Staff attending the stabilisation or resuscitation of a newborn baby must be aware that PPE can hinder communication. The pre-brief should identify if there are either members of the team or the family who have specific communication needs. Masks impacting lip reading for example has been a real problem for many people and most organisations don't provide clear masks. The people impacted find it difficult to have conversations in environments where both PPE and environmental noise are present.

Although PPE is now commonplace in the hospital setting, for members of the public it can be daunting, especially when full FFP3 respirators and PPE is required. PPE is perceived by staff as a psychological barrier for patients and in one survey expressed unease that it might cause anxiety.[472]

Aerosol generating procedures (AGPs)

For pathogens that may be transmitted by airborne transmission and, possibly, those ordinarily spread by droplets, AGPs represent a risk of transmission to the resuscitation team. Neonatal AGPs include:
- Mask ventilation (using either T-piece or self-inflating bag)
- CPAP
- Intubation
- Ventilation via a tracheal tube or laryngeal mask
- Suctioning of the airway.

Neonatal chest compressions may be an AGP but they are not listed because the baby will have always undergone one of the above interventions (all of which are AGPs) prior to the onset of chest compressions.

Manikin particle dispersal studies show reduced particle dispersal with a high efficiency particulate air (HEPA) filter in place. The filter adds a slight increased resistance to airflow which potentially could increase if the filter is wet for example with longer term use. A filter could be used with either ventilation via a mask or tracheal tube using either a T-piece or bag/valve system. If a filter is used it is important that it is an appropriate size for the baby, and does not compromise ventilation. If mask ventilating with a filter in place, care should be taken that the weight of the filter does not affect mask hold and increase mask leak.

Should parents witness the resuscitation of their newborn baby?

The European paediatric resuscitation guidelines have been supportive of parental presence during resuscitation of children since 2005 [473] but the same has not been true of any newborn resuscitation guidelines until recently. The most recent European Resuscitation Council guidelines for newborn resuscitation and support of transition of infants at birth acknowledge changing of attitudes and state

"it is reasonable for mothers/fathers/partners to be present during the resuscitation where circumstances, facilities and parental inclination allow".[1]

Although pregnancy and birth are very personal experiences that many parents enjoy, it is still common for the resuscitation of the baby, if it is required, to take place away from them; either in a separate area within the delivery room or, in some cases, in a separate room altogether. In these cases, the birth partner may be able to be present but the mother is often restricted to the bed or operating table due to ongoing interventions. The physical separation of the baby from the parents causes the parents additional anxiety and stress. Being unable to witness a resuscitation can have long-term implications for the relative; in a cluster-randomised trial of adult resuscitations being unable to be present and witness the efforts to revive a relative was associated with greater distress for at least a year after the event.[475,476]

An additional, and more recent, consideration arose during the Sars-Cov-2 virus (COVID-19) pandemic when, because the mother with suspected or proven COVID-19 infection posed an infective risk to staff, it was recommended that where possible, the resuscitation should be undertaken in a separate room or at least 2 metres away from the mother.[468,477]

Few studies examine the effect of parental presence during newborn resuscitation. Most, until recently, have concentrated on the presence or absence of the birth partner as they have usually been the only person who was able to be physically close to the resuscitation.[474] More recently, however, the use of a mother-side resuscitaire, where resuscitation takes place before the cord is clamped and cut, has allowed a unique exploration of the views of both parents and staff.[167,478,479]

A number of themes have emerged in the literature:

1. The impact of parental presence on neonatal outcomes

This aspect of parental presence was explored as part of an ILCOR CoSTR.[480] It was also explored jointly with paediatric outcomes as part of a systematic review.[481] Few data, and none from an RCT, exist and it is impossible to say whether neonatal outcomes are better or worse when the parents were present or not.

2. The potential impact of parental presence on the performance of resuscitation staff

A concern for many staff has been that the already stressful situation of a newborn resuscitation might be exacerbated due to the additional anxiety of being watched or that the parents become distressed and disrupt the process.[474,478] This does not, however, seem to be borne out and limited evidence suggests that, with increasing exposure to resuscitation incidents where the parents are present, the anxiety decreases.[474,478] In a study of tracheal intubation in the NICU setting, parental presence was more likely to occur when performed by an experienced member of staff.[482] Despite the fears that there would be the additional burden of supporting a distressed parent, the workload of the resuscitation staff does not seem to be increased by parental presence and, in babies who are healthier (as judged by higher 5 minute Apgar scores), it might actually be lower.[483]

3. The emotional and psychological impact for the parent

For parents, birth can present a rollercoaster of emotions, particularly if the baby is premature.[484] The reported reactions of parents witnessing resuscitation varies between individuals and is a mix of anxiety, anticipation and reassurance. Many parents in the study of mother-side resuscitation expressed the view that they may have been more worried had their baby been removed to a distant resuscitaire and that witnessing various resuscitation manoeuvres was beneficial to help them understand the process and that staff were doing things appropriately.[478]

4. Support for the parents and how this is best offered during resuscitation

For many parents, resuscitation is a novel experience; where resuscitation is anticipated and time permits, a pre-delivery explanation of what might happen should form part of the planning and pre-brief. The decision who should be present during any potential stabilisation of resuscitation should be agreed jointly between the resuscitation team and the parents. Some parents may not want to witness the events and, with mother-side resuscitation, this might mean adapting existing equipment to include screens if the benefits of DCC (Chapter 6) are to be retained.

Parents are likely to have questions, a running commentary might pre-empt many of these, but it may not always be possible to provide a separate and experienced healthcare professional who can facilitate this. The most experienced resuscitator may well be too busy to undertake this role.

Whether parents are present at newborn stabilisation and resuscitation varies considerably; in part the decision may be determined by the geographical location of the resuscitaire in relation to the mother. Extrapolating from studies in adults and older children would suggest that being present during resuscitation is beneficial for parents but, as yet remains poorly studied in the newborn setting.

There appears to be no good reason to exclude parents other than the physical need to move the baby to a separate area or room. Redesigning delivery rooms to allow both parents to see resuscitation events is one option but would require investment in some cases. Even with existing equipment, with a little forethought and planning, there is no good reason why there could not be a paradigm shift allowing parents to witness the stabilisation and resuscitation of their baby.

Horizon scanning

Predicting the future is difficult but there are multiple areas of active research in neonatology including areas that affect resuscitation. Areas where new information may become available include, but are not limited to: respiratory function monitoring, waveform capnography, video debriefing and parental presence at resuscitation.

A: **Summary learning**

There is still much to learn about the optimum way to assist newborn babies make the transition to breathing air.

Approaches, drugs and equipment that have been commonly used are being scrutinised to provide an evidence-based approach.

Not all evidence will come from randomised controlled trials.

Appendix B
Practical procedures

Introduction

The practical procedures covered in this appendix are technically challenging, and being practical skills, cannot be adequately taught in a manual. The indications, techniques and common complications of some of the more regularly performed practical procedures in newborn resuscitation and in neonatal intensive care are discussed here, however, the procedures themselves are best taught under direct supervision in controlled settings until competence is achieved.

Nasopharyngeal airway (NPA)

Insertion of a nasopharyngeal airway (NPA) is designed to open the channel between the nostril and the nasopharynx. As most newborns are obligate nasal breathers this technique is particularly effective in this age group. An NPA is better tolerated by a conscious baby than an oropharyngeal airway. The technique is most commonly used to support a baby who has partial upper airway obstruction with patent nasal passageways and an adequate respiratory drive. This includes babies with congenital anomalies such as micrognathia, a large tongue (macroglossia) or other pathology causing restriction of the naso- or oropharyngeal spaces.[485-487]

The NPA is a soft flexible plastic or silicone bevelled tube. Once sited the additional flange material may be cut down and used to secure the device in the correct position. There are specifically manufactured tubes for this purpose, however if these are not available a standard tracheal tube can also be used (Figure B1).

A correctly placed NPA will lie just above the epiglottis and separates the soft palate and back of the tongue from the posterior wall of the oro-pharynx. If the airway is too short it will fail to achieve this separation and if too long it can pass into the larynx and aggravate cough and gag reflexes. It is possible to estimate the length of the NPA required from the overall length of the baby[488,489] but in the emergency situation, the length can be more readily estimated by measuring the distance from the tip of the nose to the tragus of the ear. Irrespective of the method chosen, there should be a significant improvement in the patient's respiratory status if the NPA is correctly placed and this too should guide the final length.

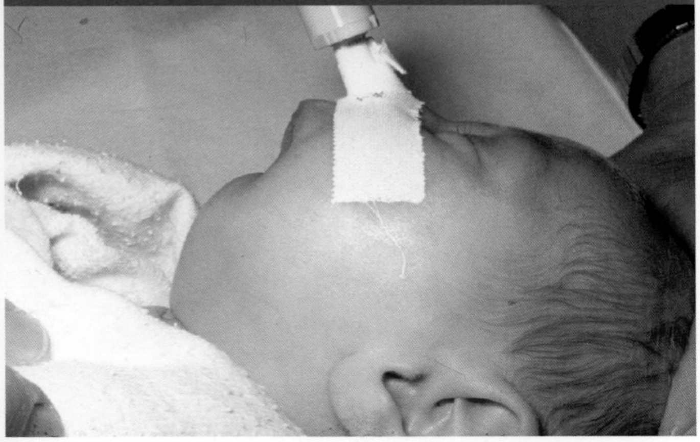

The size of the tube (diameter) can be estimated by visually matching its diameter against the internal diameter of the anterior nostril, although this is not always the narrowest part of the nasal airway and a smaller tube may be required if resistance is felt.[490]

The nasopharyngeal airway should be lubricated and introduced into the nostril with a gentle rotating motion passing the airway directly backwards and posteriorly along the floor of the nose. The length of the airway should be confirmed, if possible, by direct vision with a laryngoscope, observing that the tip of the device appears in view at the top of the oropharynx. The correct sized tube should fit snugly in the nostril without causing blanching of the nares.

This device is not suitable for infants with obstruction to the choanal space, significant coagulopathy or if there are copious or tenacious secretions.

Tracheal intubation

This manual can only discuss the practicalities of intubation. Tracheal intubation cannot be learnt from a book, a lecture or a video. Manikins currently available, even if they are 'intubatable', do not offer a completely realistic experience and the best way is to be taught on an appropriately-sized anaesthetised patient by an experienced practitioner. Tracheal intubation can be performed by first passing the tracheal tube through the mouth (oral tracheal intubation) or the nose (nasal tracheal intubation). The latter, however, is technically slightly more difficult and tends to be used more in the elective setting.

A videolaryngoscope, if available, is a useful tool to help learn intubation as it allows the trainer and trainee to see the same view (something clearly not possible with a standard laryngoscope). The trainer can offer advice during the procedure and, if recording, can play back the whole procedure for further review. Moreover, the trainee can be taught to recognise the landmarks that they need to identify when intubating by reviewing the recorded procedure.[491]

Studies have shown that trainee intubation success improves when a videolaryngoscope is used.[492,493] There are, however, subtle differences between the views obtained during conventional and videolaryngoscopy that need to be taken into account.[494]

Figure B1   A baby with Pierre Robin Sequence with a shortened tracheal tube being used as a nasopharyngeal airway

1. Why intubate?

Most babies who are apnoeic at birth respond to lung inflation and ventilation using a face mask or laryngeal mask and intubation is rarely necessary.

> Face mask ventilation is the technique of choice in newborn resuscitation. Other forms of airway control may be useful in specific circumstances.

Intubation can occasionally be essential, for example, if the larynx or trachea is blocked with inhaled material. It also provides a secure airway leaving the single-handed operator free to concentrate on other things in a prolonged resuscitation and in some preterm babies it allows for surfactant administration.

Intubation, with the correct size tube, can also make the ventilation of abnormally stiff lungs easier. Surfactant deficient lungs, or hypoplastic lungs following prolonged rupture of membranes (days or weeks), can sometimes be particularly difficult to aerate unless sustained pressures of 30 cm water or even higher are used at first.[495,496] If a preterm baby is intubated, consider giving surfactant.

When emergency intubation is necessary, it can be assumed, in most cases, that the baby is already limp, unresponsive and unconscious. Tracheal intubation in such circumstances is usually not difficult, although it is not a skill that staff should be expected to display without prior supervised experience as the laryngoscope blade can cause damage to the larynx.[324]

> It should be possible to place a tracheal tube within 30 s. If you fail to do so, revert to mask inflation before trying again.

It can be helpful for a second person to check how long the procedure is taking and alert the operator if it is taking too long.[497] If tracheal intubation is proving difficult then managing the airway with face mask ventilation, possibly with a two-handed jaw thrust, laryngeal mask or oropharyngeal airway, ensuring good oxygenation and calling for additional help is important.

2. Tube size and length

Use the largest suitable tracheal tube, a snug, but not tight fit, is important. Too small a tube may not allow you to aerate the lungs especially if they are stiff or full of fluid (as at birth). If the tube is too small, gas will escape through the gap between the tube and the tracheal wall. If the lungs are at all stiff, so much gas will escape through the leak that the lungs will not be inflated sufficiently. This can easily be detected by listening at the mouth or over the neck with a stethoscope while inflating the lung. Bubbles may appear at the mouth and chest movement will be poor. If you have chosen the right size tube and you can hear a large air-leak you may have intubated the oesophagus.

Tracheal tubes are classified by their internal diameter (ID) in millimetres. Tubes from different manufacturers may have different wall thicknesses and though it is the internal diameter that is most important from the respiratory point of view, it is the outside diameter that determines whether the tube will fit snugly into the larynx of any particular baby. For example, 2.5 mm tubes can vary in external diameter from 3.5 to 4.1 mm and similar variations occur in other sizes.[498] Most manufacturers also mark their tubes a certain distance from the tip, however these vary considerably between manufacturers.[499]

Whilst formulae can give an estimate of the length of the tube, these can be unreliable.[500] In most cases, the length and size of tracheal tube can be estimated from the gestation at birth (Table B1).[501]

3. The procedure of laryngoscopic intubation

Skilled emergency intubation depends on the prior acquisition of good technique. Develop a standard, planned and structured approach from the start. Many have found the following approach useful:

- Position all the equipment you need close by and prepare a means of securing the tracheal tube once it is in place.

- Position the baby on a firm flat working surface with the neck partially extended. A roll of blanket under the baby's shoulders may help. Do not over-extend the neck as this will stretch the trachea and position the larynx very anteriorly, making it more difficult to see and making it difficult to push the laryngeal opening into full view using external pressure on the larynx.

- Position the laryngoscope. Hold the handle in your left hand while opening the baby's mouth. While looking down the laryngoscope insert it gently into the mouth. Be careful not to damage the gums.

Table B1	A guide to tracheal tubes sizes and approximate lengths for oral and nasal intubation (adapted from Kempley et al[501])			
Gestation	Birth weight	Size*	Oral length	Nasal length
25 weeks	650 g	2.5 mm	6.0 cm	7.0 cm
28 weeks	1200 g	2.5 mm	7.0 cm	8.0 cm
31 weeks	1600 g	2.5 / 3.0 mm	7.5 cm	8.5 cm
34 weeks	2400 g	3.0 mm	8.0 cm	9.0 cm
37 weeks	3000 g	3.0 mm	9.0 cm	10.5 cm
40 weeks	3500 g	3.5 mm	9.5 cm	11.0 cm
* size means internal diameter (ID); the external diameter varies between manufacturers				

- Position the tongue. In children (and adults) the usual approach is to insert the blade into the right-hand side of the mouth (as you see it) and then to sweep the tongue to the left by bringing the blade across into the centre. In newborn babies the tongue is usually relatively fixed in the floor of the mouth and it can be easier simply to slip the blade down centrally into the mouth over the tongue.

- Position the baby (and yourself) so you can see comfortably down the laryngoscope. If the surface the baby is on is height-adjustable consider whether they are at the right height for you.

- If the laryngoscope blade is pushed in too far, all you will see is the oesophagus (Figure B2a), you then have to withdraw the blade slightly to allow the larynx to drop into view from above (Figure B2b). Alternatively, if the blade is not in far enough, you may see little except the epiglottis (Figure B2c).

- Position the larynx. Once you have found the epiglottis, placing the tip of the blade at the base of the epiglottis where it meets the tongue (the glosso-epiglottic fold and the valleculae to either side) will bring the larynx into view from behind it (Figure B2d). Slight external downward pressure on the larynx may then help to bring the laryngeal opening into the centre of the field of view (Figure B2e).

- Position the tube. Bringing the tip in from the right-hand corner of the mouth and keeping the curve of the tube horizontal so you don't obscure your view of the larynx (Figure B2f). A stylet is usually unnecessary if you have everything properly lined up but may be helpful if it is difficult to direct the tip of the tube into the laryngeal inlet. When using a stylet, do not let the tip of this extend beyond the end of the tracheal tube. If the cords are tightly adducted, wait for them to relax, don't prod as you might cause a reflex adduction of the vocal cords. Reflex cord adduction proves that the baby cannot be in terminal apnoea.

- Insert the tube 1–2 cm through the cords and no further. The vocal cord guide marks (based on measurements in human babies [502]) will help to judge this. However, it is important to remember that the distance between the tip and the mark can vary according to the manufacturer and the internal diameter of the tube.[499]

- The baby's airway is a tube, not a hole. Inserting a tracheal tube is passing one tube into another; not a tube through a hole. Try to ensure the tracheal tube is aligned with the airway otherwise it may be difficult to pass and may traumatise the fragile mucosa of the airway. This is especially important if using a stylet which makes the tube more rigid.

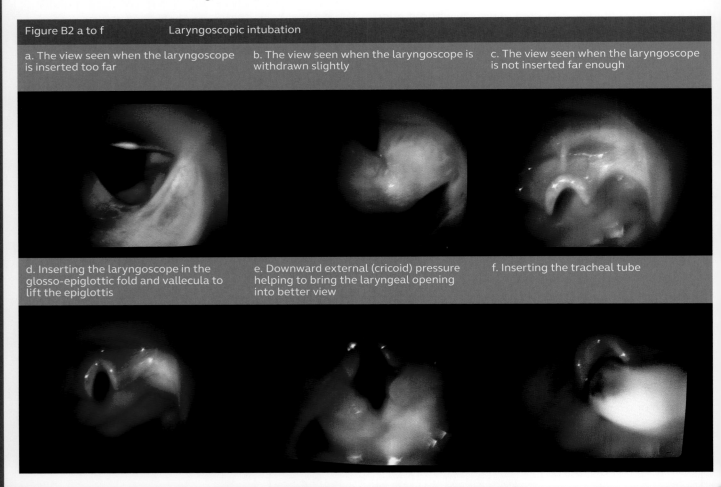

Figure B2 a to f   Laryngoscopic intubation

a. The view seen when the laryngoscope is inserted too far

b. The view seen when the laryngoscope is withdrawn slightly

c. The view seen when the laryngoscope is not inserted far enough

d. Inserting the laryngoscope in the glosso-epiglottic fold and vallecula to lift the epiglottis

e. Downward external (cricoid) pressure helping to bring the laryngeal opening into better view

f. Inserting the tracheal tube

- Once the tube is passed, gently remove the laryngoscope. The tube can be held in place against the hard palate by an index finger placed gently in the mouth.

- Aerate the lungs, with five inflation breaths if the lungs have not yet been inflated. If possible, use a controlled inflation pressure of no more than 30 cm water (25 cm water in preterm babies) sustained for 2–3 s, checking that the chest moves symmetrically. Use capnography to confirm tube placement.

- Secure the tube once you have confirmed it is correctly placed. Note the distance inserted by noting the markings at the lips. Be careful, it is easy to allow the tube to go down too far. If you do, you risk ventilating only one lung. Continue ventilating the lungs using a controlled inflation pressure checking that the chest moves symmetrically.

4. Confirming tube placement

Rapid confirmation of correct tracheal tube placement at the point of care is important because tube malposition can be associated with serious adverse outcomes, including hypoxaemia, pneumothorax, lung collapse and death.

After intubation, check that the tube is in the trachea by:
- checking the heart rate – is it increasing?[196]
- checking that the exhaled CO_2 detector confirms intubation[503]
- listen at the mouth – is there a large and audible leak?
- look at the chest – are both sides moving equally?[504]
- listen to both sides of the chest including the axillae, is air entry equal?[504]

If the tube is in the right place, the chest will normally move symmetrically as pressure is applied, and the heart rate will usually start to improve within about 30 s.

A chest x-ray should be obtained to confirm tube tip position once the baby is in the NNU; the fact that confirmatory action occurs at a time after resuscitation underlines the importance of clinical and capnography assessment.

Colorimetric CO_2 detectors

Studies suggest that detection of exhaled CO_2 confirms tracheal intubation in neonates with cardiac output more rapidly and accurately than clinical assessment alone.[505,506] Colorimetric CO_2 detectors can be used in any size baby however they may be slower to respond in very small babies due to their smaller tidal volumes. Nonetheless, use of an exhaled CO_2 detector is recommended as one of the essential checks of tube placement after a baby has been intubated.

Though capable of a very quick response,[507] there are limitations to the use of these devices:

- One can be misled about a correctly placed tube if the cardiac output is so low (i.e. significant bradycardia or asystole) then a colorimetric CO_2 detector will be negative even if the tracheal tube is correctly sited as there is insufficient CO_2 entering the baby's lungs.[507]

- Liquids spilt on the detector, such as adrenaline, surfactant or gastric contents, can cause a colour change, thus falsely suggesting that the tube is correctly placed. This may be detected as a constant colour change, whereas with a correctly placed tracheal tube there should be variation in the colour during the respiratory cycle.[508]

- Intubation of the right main bronchus will also produce a positive result, however the tip of the tracheal tube is not in the correct place.[508] Do not rely solely on the exhaled CO_2 detector and use the other checks described previously in the section 'Checking tube placement'.

- Large airway leaks may decrease tidal volume delivered to the detector which can limit the accuracy of the CO_2 detector.

- If the trachea is blocked below the tracheal tube there will be no colour change. If you are certain that the tube was correctly placed (i.e. definitely seen to pass through the cords or has been checked by a second person) then you should concentrate on clearing the tracheal blockage. Re-evaluate if there is no improvement after suctioning.

Using a colorimetric CO_2 detector

Before starting, match the initial colour of the indicator to the colour labelled 'check' around the detector window as shown in Figure B3a. If the colour of the indicator is different or darker than the area marked 'check', do not use.

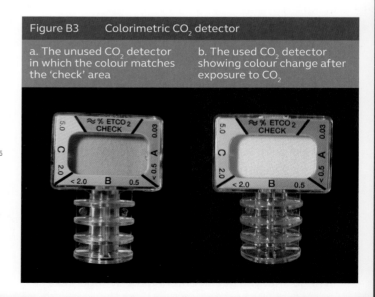

Figure B3	Colorimetric CO_2 detector
a. The unused CO_2 detector in which the colour matches the 'check' area	b. The used CO_2 detector showing colour change after exposure to CO_2

- Intubate the patient.

- Firmly attach the CO_2 detector to the tracheal tube, then attach the breathing device and ventilate the patient with six breaths of moderate tidal volume.

- Compare the indicator colour in the window on full-end expiration to ranges printed on the detector cover. A correctly placed tube will result in a colour change that fluctuates between the check and CO_2 detection colours (purple/yellow (Figure B3b).

- If the results are negative or not conclusive, use clinical assessment to check tube placement. Remove the tube if this assessment suggests incorrect placement.

- An intermediate colour change (without variation) may occur in an oesophageal intubation due to retained CO_2 in the oesophagus or in a correctly placed tube if the baby is already hypocarbic (i.e. over-ventilated).

Emergency needle thoracocentesis

Needle aspiration (thoracocentesis) is an immediate intervention used in cases of tension pneumothorax where there is evidence of cardiorespiratory compromise. Signs of a pneumothorax include unequal chest movement, respiratory compromise, tachycardia followed by bradycardia and occasionally a displaced mediastinum. Pneumothorax can be confirmed using transillumination in small, usually preterm, babies but the thickness of the skin and thoracic walls, along with the lighting levels in a delivery suite, make this less effective in term babies.

There is usually insufficient time to obtain x-ray confirmation of a life-threatening tension pneumothorax, thus the diagnosis is a clinical one. There is, however, a 10–20% chance of causing a pneumothorax if thoracocentesis is attempted and the baby **does not** have a pneumothorax, thus the procedure should not be undertaken lightly.

- Clean the skin quickly using alcohol wipes. Allow the alcohol to dry before proceeding.

- Identify the site of insertion (this is the second intercostal space in the mid-clavicular line) by palpating the infant's sternum to find the manubriosternal angle (or angle of Louis). This marks the approximate level of the second pair of costal cartilages, which, in turn, attach to the second ribs. Follow the ribs along the side of the pneumothorax to the mid-point between both ends of the clavicle.

- Insert a 22G butterfly needle or cannula into the second intercostal space (i.e. below the second rib and aiming just above the third rib) perpendicular to the chest. Inserting the needle just above the third rib avoids the neurovascular bundles that run along the lower borders of each of the ribs.

- As you insert the needle/cannula aspirate with a syringe until you get air entering the syringe. Take

care not to damage the underlying lung by advancing the needle and carefully aspirating as you go. Stop advancing as soon as you aspirate air or there is a clinical improvement. Once you cannot aspirate any more air remove the needle to prevent injury to the lung.

- Alternatively, if you are using a butterfly needle the end of this can be held under water (e.g. larger ampoules of 0.9% sodium chloride or water for injection may be the most conveniently available). The entrapped air will bubble through confirming correct placement.

- Once stabilised consider insertion of a formal chest drain.

Umbilical vein catheterisation

Umbilical vein catheterisation is the most commonly used, and preferred, method for obtaining venous access in the newborn baby; intraosseous needles may be an alternative outside labour wards.

When to consider umbilical vein catheterisation

If the heart rate is still not improving despite good lung aeration, ventilation and a period of chest compressions, then drugs or volume may be considered. Although umbilical vein catheterisation is seldom necessary in the emergency resuscitation of a newborn baby, it is also a quick and effective way to gain access to the central circulation in a baby who has collapsed for several days after birth.[509]

It can be critically important to be able to give volume replacement or drugs, to transfuse a baby, or useful to sample blood from a baby who is peripherally 'shut down'. Trying to cannulate a peripheral vein is more difficult, slower and most importantly, will be ineffective for delivering drugs to the heart when the circulation is absent.

Equipment

Immediate access to a sterile pack containing all the essential equipment makes rapid and reliable umbilical catheterisation much easier. A basic pack could usefully contain:

- scalpel and a straight edged blade (e.g. No 11)

- 5 French gauge end-hole umbilical catheter

- three-way tap and 5 mL syringe

- two artery forceps

- one umbilical vein probe (may be helpful, not essential)

- some sterile gauze squares, a cord ligature or tape.

If this is a real emergency, there is no time for full aseptic technique; however you and an assistant should wear sterile gloves and observe universal precautions for your own safety.

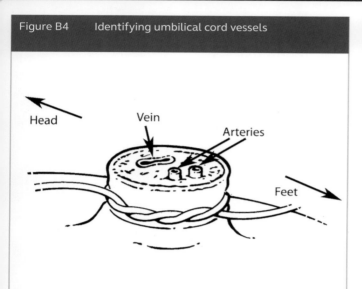

Figure B4   Identifying umbilical cord vessels

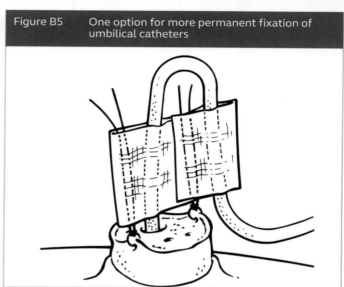

Figure B5   One option for more permanent fixation of umbilical catheters

Technique

Prepare the equipment. Fill a 5 mL syringe with 0.9% sodium chloride and flush through a three-way tap attached to the umbilical catheter. Turn the tap to occlude the catheter to prevent air being sucked into the circulation should the baby gasp. Before you take a blood sample you have to aspirate back all the flush solution and a further 2–3 mL of blood to ensure there is no contamination of the sample for testing.

- Tie the cord ligature or tape loosely around the base of the cord. If a second twist is added to the tie (Figure B4) then it will hold if it is necessary later to pull it tight. The arteries are unlikely to bleed though bleeding from the vein is likely. However, arterial bleeding may follow recovery.

- Cut the cord 1–2 cm from the skin with a clean stroke of the scalpel. A sawing action results in a rough cut edge of the umbilical cord making catheterisation more difficult.

- Identify the umbilical vessels (Figure B4). There are usually two arteries and one vein; occasionally only a single artery is present. The vein travels 'north' (i.e. superiorly) from the umbilicus as the ductus venosus immediately beneath the anterior abdominal wall, passing through the liver to join the hepatic and portal veins then joining the inferior vena cava and entering the right atrium. The arteries are branches of the iliac vessels and enter the umbilicus from the 'south' (i.e. inferiorly). When the cord is cut close to the skin the thin-walled vein is usually found somewhere in the upper right quadrant, while the two stiff, string-like, white and bloodless contracted arteries are usually found somewhere in the two lower quadrants. Be sure to identify all three vessels.

- Grasp the cord with the artery forceps near the vein. Gently insert the catheter into the vein using fingers

or forceps. Do not probe the vein without supporting it by its edge with forceps. The umbilical vein may need to be gently dilated using a probe or a closed artery forceps but is often easily entered without this.

- Advance the catheter until some resistance is felt at the umbilical ring just below the skin. Apply gentle pressure until the catheter passes through. The ideal place for the end of the catheter is within the inferior vena cava just outside the right atrium. In an emergency it is sufficient to get the end of the catheter in a large vessel – in other words into a vessel from which it is easy to aspirate blood. In the typical (3.5 kg) term baby, a correctly placed UVC is inserted to 10–11 cm (plus the length of the cord).

- Draw back on the syringe and blood should flow back if the catheter is in the right place. If blood is not drawn back easily insert the catheter a little further or withdraw it slightly and try again. The first sample of blood can usefully be sent for pH, blood gases and haematocrit estimation.

- Flush the catheter gently with 0.9% sodium chloride when in the right place to avoid thrombosis in the catheter.

- Secure the catheter. In an emergency, tape the catheter in place with one piece of tape across the abdomen. One of a number of methods for more permanent fixation is shown in Figure B5.

- Give drugs and volume replacement with O Rh(D) negative blood or 0.9% sodium chloride if required.

- Whenever possible, umbilical catheterisation is best undertaken as a sterile procedure, in a properly equipped, warm, treatment area after the airway has been secured, and the circulation restored. It is also worth considering using a double-lumen umbilical catheter in such circumstances.

Securing an umbilical catheter

On the very rare occasions when this is needed as an emergency at delivery, it almost always involves a term or near-term baby. Under these circumstances the priority is to secure the UVC as central venous access. This can be done by taping the catheter securely to the abdomen.

If there is more time, one simple way to secure an umbilical catheter is to put two silk stitches into the substance of the umbilical cord, tie these in place and cut them about two inches long (Figure B5). Line these ends up alongside the catheter, turn the catheter back on itself and tape all together such that the catheter is taped to the silk. The catheter is then held securely in place with no tape attached to the skin. If it is necessary to adjust the catheter length after checking the position of the tip by X-ray or ultrasound this can be easily done.

Insertion of an intraosseous needle

Intraosseous needles have been used as emergency access in the event of failed peripheral, central and umbilical venous access in infants since 1943.[510] The technique was largely abandoned during the 1950s through to the 1980, with the introduction of plastic catheters that allowed more prolonged vascular access.[511]

Intraosseous needles are not commonly used in neonatal intensive care or in newborn resuscitation, but nonetheless can provide rapid central access through which both resuscitation drugs and emergency fluids can be administered[437] In simulated newborn resuscitations they can be inserted as quickly as an umbilical venous catheter.[437,512] A number of complications have been associated with newborn use of IO.[270] However, the intraosseous route may also be useful in the very rare situation when a baby who needs drugs during resuscitation but has an abnormal looking umbilical cord or a congenital abnormality (such as an abdominal wall defect) where UVC cannot be inserted or is in the ED or out-of-hospital situation where practitioners may be less used to umbilical catheterisation.[271]

Insertion technique

- There are different types of intraosseous needles; newer types are inserted using an automatic 'drill'.
- Identify the insertion point on the anteromedial surface of the tibia, just below the tibial tuberosity.
- Insert the needle applying downwards pressure until a 'give' is felt and the needle enters the bone marrow cavity.
- Take any samples needed (notify the laboratory that they are bone marrow samples as the high white cell count in a sample can be mistaken for leukaemia). Prioritise important tests from these samples such as glucose and cultures.

Complications and considerations

- complications are rare but can be potentially serious[513,514]
- intraosseous needles should not be used if the bone is abnormal (e.g. osteogenesis imperfecta)
- there is risk of fracture to the bone particularly in small babies[515]
- bone marrow embolism has been described.

Despite the ease of insertion of intraosseous needles, umbilical venous access remains the emergency vascular access procedure of choice on delivery suite.

A: **Summary learning**

Practical skills discussed in this appendix are how to:
- secure an airway using nasopharyngeal airway insertion or tracheal intubation
- drain a life-threatening tension pneumothorax
- obtain vascular access using umbilical venous catheterisation or intraosseous needle insertion.

These important skills are not needed in most newborn resuscitations.

These skills should only be undertaken by personnel who have been trained in these techniques and who are deemed competent to do so.

Introduction

The basic principles which underwrite the approach to resuscitation at birth have evolved over the years through an incremental process and the same applies to the equipment used. The basic requirements are broadly very similar to those initially described in the 1960s when much of the approach to resuscitation we now take as standard was being developed.

There is some value in reflecting on how the approach we adopt reflects the available technology. Large parts of the world lack the abundance of resources available in the National Health Service; how to deliver high-quality stabilisation and resuscitation in a resource-limited setting reminds us how much can be achieved with relatively little equipment – providing it is used to good effect by people trained in its use.

Thermal care

For babies who are healthy, the natural warmth of their mother is the best means of keeping warm as well as helping bonding. Delivering the baby onto the abdomen, then drying and wrapping it in such a way as to maintain skin-to-skin contact helps. Such an approach is equally valid for the late preterm baby who, following assessment, ideally with the umbilical cord intact, is felt to be coping with breathing. Out-of-hospital, this is a valid means of supporting babies during their transfer to hospital at all gestations, providing airway and breathing can be maintained.

Should it be necessary to separate mother and baby for the purposes of assessment, stabilisation or resuscitation then consideration of the environment is vital. Modifying external factors such as using heaters, closing windows and minimising draughts is important. Operating theatres, for example, are frequently not optimised for the thermal needs of the baby who is about to be delivered. It can be a challenge to get the temperature pushed high enough, especially if the baby is < 28 weeks gestation when an ambient temperature greater than 26°C is required.[215] The same principles apply to any delivery area, whether this is in a hospital or not. It is important that you should be proactive on behalf of the baby.

Drying and wrapping is a tried and tested method of keeping babies warm that reduces convective and evaporative losses. It requires no more than two towels, and whilst a radiant heater is helpful it may not be necessary for the mature, unstressed baby if the ambient temperature is appropriate. It is only when exposed that additional adjuncts are needed.

In preterm babies, placing them undried into a plastic bag and providing an external heat source creates an optimal thermal environment. In situations where a radiant source is not available but additional heat is required, an exothermic mattress can be used.[516,517] Exothermic mattresses are also useful during transfers but if using care must be taken to avoid direct contact of the baby with it. This is also true for other unregulated heat sources such as hot water bottles. If using multiple heat sources, be careful not to overheat the baby.

Resuscitaires (and other working surfaces)

The ideal working area for newborn resuscitation is a flat, non-slip surface that is firm, but cushioned, and insulated to prevent heat loss. Some platforms have offered active warming, but this is not required in general.

The surface should be at a height that permits unhindered intervention. The floor may be the best surface in the community. Many resuscitaires now have height-adjustable platforms, but remember that one height may not suit all members of the team. A pre-requisite for effective intervention is to be able see what is going on so having adequate lighting is important.

Recent developments have promoted initial assessment of the baby near the mother with delayed cord clamping (DCC) ongoing. In recognition of this a number of devices have been developed which permit support of transition and even resuscitation beside the mother, with bedside platforms (Figure C1) providing all the facilities of traditional resuscitaires.[172,518] The benefits of DCC are discussed in Chapter 6.

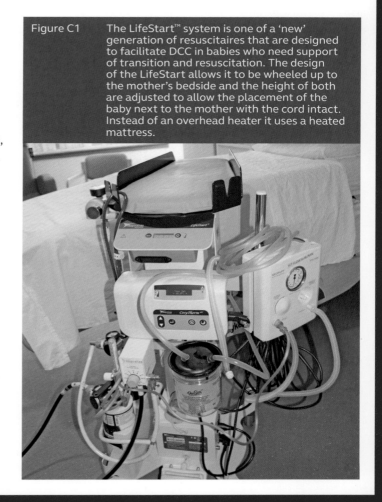

| Figure C1 | The LifeStart™ system is one of a 'new' generation of resuscitaires that are designed to facilitate DCC in babies who need support of transition and resuscitation. The design of the LifeStart allows it to be wheeled up to the mother's bedside and the height of both are adjusted to allow the placement of the baby next to the mother with the cord intact. Instead of an overhead heater it uses a heated mattress. |

Delivering inflation and ventilation breaths

1. T-pieces

The T-piece can only function if connected to a regulated positive pressure gas supply. Systems permit regulation of the flow of gas through the T-piece, the concentration of oxygen via a blender and the pressure delivered. Most, but not all, T-pieces allow variation in the peak inspiratory pressure (PIP) and the level of positive end expiratory pressure (PEEP) through adjustable relief valves on the system, or the T-piece itself. Most systems have a secondary safety blow off valve, this is usually set to somewhere between 30 and 40 cm water. This is a safety feature that does not normally need adjusting however, it will need to be altered if higher pressures are required.

When setting up a T-piece circuit it is important to check the level of PEEP and PIP before use. Flows of 5–8 L min^{-1} are typical of those required. Some circuits are supplied with the PEEP valve screwed shut in which case potentially dangerous levels of pressure may be delivered to the baby if used unchecked. PEEP is flow rate dependent and if the flow rate is changed, then the delivered PEEP will also change.[519-521]

Flow is also important in determining tidal volume when the lungs are inflated. Pressure is used as a proxy for tidal volume in the inflation and ventilation of babies, but it is not the only factor to take into consideration.

Pressure is the driving force that allows the delivery of a given volume by overcoming the opening pressure in the lung. Once the lung is opened, the pressure, the inspiratory time and the flow rate are variables which determine the actual tidal volume delivered.

This can be illustrated simply by the following example: A 0.5 second inspiratory breath when using a T-piece (and when there is minimal leak) at 6 L min^{-1} will deliver 50 mL per breath. This is higher than the 17–25 mL tidal volumes in term babies (assuming a normal tidal volume of 4–8 mL kg^{-1}). This is also much higher than the tidal volumes of a preterm baby.

It is vital that the T-piece system is connected to a regulated (and therefore pressure-limited) supply, not direct to 'wall' oxygen which could result in dangerously high pressures and gas volumes being delivered. Whilst historically this may have been possible, this is unlikely to happen with current resuscitation equipment if it is used correctly.

Whilst effective ventilation of the newborn can be achieved with a flow-inflating bag (not very common in a newborn setting in the UK), a self-inflating bag or with a pressure limited T-piece resuscitator.[522,523] The advantages of the T-piece are:

- For most people, it is easier to use than a self-inflating bag and mask, especially for the single-handed resuscitator.[188,524]

- It has the ability to deliver adjustable PEEP through the screw valve on the circuit (Figure C3).[522]

- In use, the T-piece delivers a more constant peak pressure for an operator-determined time interval. [522,525]

There are some disadvantages; the T-piece system requires a gas supply and thus cannot be used in situations where this is unavailable. Users of T-pieces are less able to detect changes in compliance as users of either self-inflating or flow-inflating bags.[526]

T-pieces may be device specific or generic. Care needs to be taken as there are different fittings to enable connection to the gas supply. Some use the generic 15 mm connector; others have bespoke, narrower fittings requiring an adaptor.

2. Self-inflating bags

Self-inflating bags provide gas under pressure in the absence of an external, pressurised supply. They are, therefore, useful in situations when such a gas supply is not available, in which case the inspired gas will be air. They can be used with an oxygen supply, allowing the inspired gas mixture to approach oxygen concentrations up to 90% if a rebreathing bag is connected.

The appropriate tidal volume during resuscitation is not known, most studies concentrate on establishing an adequate functional residual capacity (FRC)[95] and so we have to extrapolate from experience with spontaneously breathing babies at birth, ventilated babies after birth, and animal studies. For ventilated babies, with aerated lungs, a tidal volume of 4–8 mL kg^{-1}, at a rate of 40–60, provides adequate control of the partial pressure of CO_2.[527]

During the first inflations, where the fluid is moved out of the airways and an FRC is being developed, tidal volumes may need to be larger. Studies of colorimetric exhaled CO_2 detection and respiratory function, have shown that if the tidal volume is < 3.2 mL kg^{-1} then exhaled CO_2 may

Figure C3   Two types of T-piece with adjustable screw-type PEEP valves.

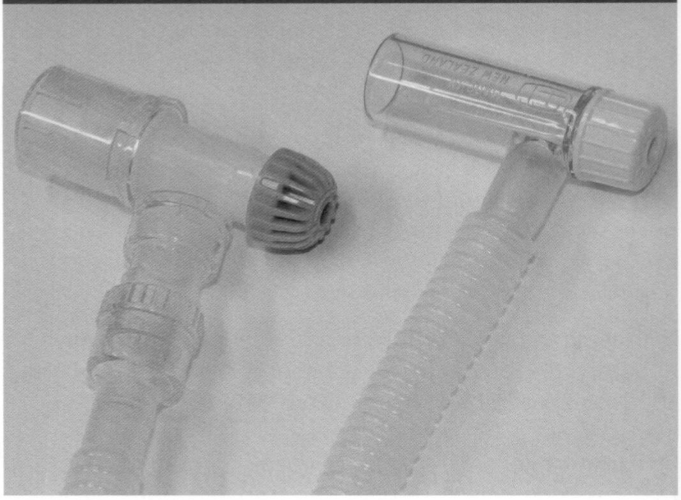

not be detected.[528] The tidal volumes for spontaneously breathing newborn preterm infants, however, ranged from 4.2 to 5.8 mL kg^{-1} when receiving CPAP.[321]

Despite our lack of knowledge of the appropriate tidal volume for the first few breaths of the newborn baby it is certainly less than the 500 mL that is the recommended size bag for resuscitation at birth. Bags are available in smaller sizes (e.g. 240 mL) but these may make it difficult to achieve the 2–3 s duration of pressure required for inflation breaths. Using the 500 mL self-inflating bag in more measured fashion allows the user to transition to the shorter ventilation breaths when the lungs have been inflated.[529]

There are many different types of self-inflating bags. Some are single-patient use only, others require sterilisation between patents. Those used for paediatric and neonatal purposes usually have a pressure-relief valve in the circuit. This must be tested before use by occluding the bag outlet and squeezing. Once the pressure in the bag exceeds the blow-off pressure, the valve should open and flow be heard.

The blow-off valve is usually a spring mechanism set at a pressure between 30 and 40 cm water. When the bag is squeezed vigorously, the valve will not prevent excess pressure/volume being delivered to the baby – in this case the inertia of the valve is such that a higher pressure may inadvertently be given for a short period of time.[530]

> Always test the blow-off valve before using a self-inflating bag

Seal the outlet to the baby and squeeze the bag (Figure C4). You should hear the blow-off valve working as the pressure rises, if you do not hear this, check the valve mechanism. The valve may be broken or faulty[531] or, in rare cases, be missing altogether if the self-inflating bag is assembled using the connector from an adult bag.[532]

In use, the bag should be squeezed gently to achieve a pressure of about 30 cm water and sustained for 2–3 s. If the blow off valve is pre-set to 35–40 cm water (depending on the manufacturer), then activation of the valve will provide an indication that this pressure has been exceeded. Continued squeezing to just keep the valve open will allow delivery of a sustained inflation breath at the pre-set pressure. Aggressive squeezing will deliver higher pressures and excessive flow.[530]

On rare occasions, such as when faced with difficult to inflate, stiff lungs in the mature baby, pressures in excess of the blow-off valve may be required. The blow-off valve can be over-ridden by preventing the valve opening by pressing on the valve (or, in some cases, screwing it shut). Care must be taken in these circumstances as unless there is some other means of monitoring the pressure there is no way to know the actual pressure being delivered. Once the lungs have been inflated using these higher

pressures every consideration should be given to reducing these pressures as long as the heart rate is maintained and chest movement is seen.

Most self-inflating bags come with some form of oxygen reservoir (this can be a reservoir bag or additional tubing; with re-useable devices this is also usually detachable). If you are using air alone, this is a redundant device but when used with an oxygen supply this can allow the delivery of > 90% oxygen because when the squeezed portion of the self-inflating bag re-inflates it draws oxygen from the source and from the reservoir.[216]

If the reservoir bag is not used, but an oxygen supply remains connected, when the squeezed portion of the self-inflating bag re-inflates it will draw in air from the atmosphere and the system will deliver between 30–70% oxygen depending on the flow rate of oxygen.[214,215] It is impossible to be precise about the amount of oxygen in these situations as there is no calibration.

The design of the self-inflating bag makes it cumbersome for the single person to use. The self-inflating bag is at 90° to the direction of force required to make a good face mask seal, thus the mechanics work against the operator in maintaining that seal. There are newer designs of self-inflating bag for neonatal use which have a simpler design with the bag oriented vertically, making it easier to hold and maintain an even pressure on the mask (Figure C5). These systems have been designed for use in health care systems where oxygen is not available and do not have a reservoir.

3. Gas supply

Current evidence supports starting resuscitation of term infants using air. Supplemental oxygen is rarely needed. In the UK hospital setting all delivery areas will have piped, pressurised ('wall') oxygen and it is not unusual to have piped, pressurised air. In low-risk birth centres, resuscitaires may run off cylinder gas. In these cases,

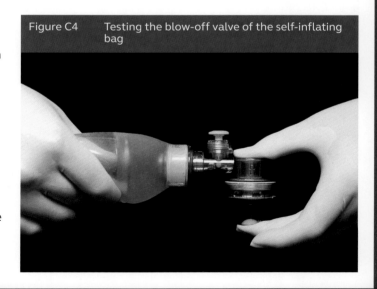

Figure C4 Testing the blow-off valve of the self-inflating bag

it is essential that the pre-birth check ensures that the cylinders are able to continue throughout even the most complex resuscitation and subsequent care pending a transfer.

In most UK community settings, and in low resource settings, piped or cylinder gas is not usually available. If it is, it is usually oxygen, not air. Blended mixtures, therefore, are rarely used but a self-inflating bag may permit some variation in the delivered oxygen concentration.

Flow rates of approximately 5 to 8 L min[-1] are sufficient for the majority of interventions depending on the device in use. The compliance of the baby's lungs will modify the rate at which the peak pressure is achieved.

With non-invasive support, and significant soft-tissue dead space, the high compliance of the soft tissues buffers the low compliance of the lungs to slow the rate of pressure rise. When intubated this effect is removed, and the stiff lungs enable the peak pressure to be achieved very rapidly with potential risks. In this case, lower flow rates might suffice. Pressure delivery to the lungs is greater when intubated compared to non-invasive ventilation (e.g. mask ventilation). This should be considered when setting inspired pressures. Pressure delivery is reduced by mask leak or leak around a tracheal tube.

Where possible (and especially in the case of preterm babies < 32 weeks gestation) heated humidified gases should be used. These have a beneficial effect on admission temperatures in preterm babies, which are related to deceased mortality, but it is not clear if this translates into improvements in other outcomes.[533-535]

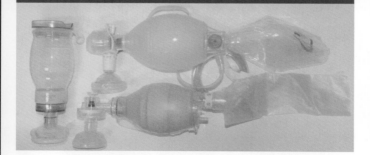

Figure B5   A selection of self-inflating bags.

From left to right; a vertically-aligned, 'in line' self-inflating bag without reservoir – this has a smaller bladder and new design of mask with flange; (top) a single-use 500 mL bag with fixed reservoir and valve with an override mechanism; and (bottom) a traditional self-inflating bag with removable reservoir.

Assessing heart rate

1. Stethoscopes

Listening to the heart rate using a stethoscope is an inexpensive and simple way of assessing heart rate. In low-risk babies, it can provide a reasonably accurate estimate of heart rate in about 15 seconds[536] but compared to pulse oximetry and ECG, will underestimate heart rate.[536,537]

If a stethoscope is not available it may be possible to assess the heart rate by feeling for a pulse in the umbilical cord stump, brachial or femoral arteries or by observing or feeling the pulsation of the ventricle against the chest wall. These techniques are only reliable if the heart rate is fast (> 100 min[-1]). There is a tendency for them to be inaccurate, intermittent and affected by movements. In most cases there is a significant underestimate of the heart rate that may potentially prompt inappropriate interventions.[39,538] Therefore, these methods should only be used when no alternatives exist.

2.   Pulse oximetry

Pulse oximetry gives a quick and relatively accurate display, of both heart rate and oxygen saturation, and one that easily seen by all involved in the resuscitation. This is particularly useful when stabilising significantly preterm babies or when tempted to give additional oxygen to any baby.

The pulse oximeter probe should be fitted preferentially to the right hand or wrist as this will give pre-ductal oxygen saturation values. However, fitting the probe takes time and the machine also needs to boot-up before it can start to give information. With practice, reliable data can be obtained within 60–90 s of delivery.[539] In most cases, placing a saturation probe and starting the saturation monitor depends on the arrival of a second person; until that second person arrives the priority is to deliver good quality basic life support as per the NLS algorithm.

Studies differ whether any advantage is gained from connecting the sensor to infant[539] or oximeter first,[131] however signal acquisition can be achieved within about 15 s once connected.

Once the pulse rate is displayed it is likely that this will be more accurate than listening with a stethoscope[536] and in many instances as accurate as ECG monitoring.[537] Pulse oximetry can sometimes significantly underestimate the heart rate when the signal quality is poor.[540] Peripheral hypoperfusion, signal dropout, movement, arrhythmias, and ambient lighting can all impact on signal quality.

3. ECG monitoring

There is an increasing evidence base supporting the use of ECG monitoring as a means of rapidly determining the heart rate during resuscitation.[541,542] At least two studies suggest that it may be faster than pulse oximetry.[129,543] The ability to generate an ECG is determined by the ability to reliably place electrodes on the baby as well as by having necessary monitoring equipment in place at the right time.

This has the advantage of giving an immediate indication of heart rate without delay providing the electrodes maintain effective skin contact. Compared to pulse oximetry it more readily detects bradycardia and allows an earlier intervention.[544]

The ECG, however, indicates only the electrical rate of the heart, it provides no information on the effectiveness of any contractions. Just because there is an electrical heart rhythm does not mean the heart is pumping effectively and chest compressions might still be necessary.[130,545]

It is, therefore, important to understand the limitations of any method of assessing heart rate.

Suction

It is unusual for the airway to be blocked due to secretions, blood, vernix or meconium, and thus for suction to be routinely required. However, the ability to clear an obstructed airway is essential whether it is in a hospital setting with wall suction, or in the community where portable devices need to be used.[546]

Whichever systems are used, it is vital that the suction catheter is of sufficient calibre to enable removal of thick particulate material, which is more likely to cause a problem than thin watery secretions. It is recommended that suction take place under direct vision in order to prevent inadvertent trauma to the airway or stimulation of the pharynx leading to gagging and/or vagus nerve-induced bradycardia.[547,548]

There are two types of suction catheter; rigid 'Yankauer' catheters, and longer, flexible catheters (Figures C6 and C7). Any catheter narrower than 12 French gauge is unlikely to be effective during resuscitation. Yankauer catheters have the potential advantage of a wider orifice, and can be directed with more precision but are rigid and thus need to be used with care. Their shorter length and tapered design means that they are better able to cope with thick material than the long polyurethane catheters which will rapidly block as the length of tubing the material has to pass up is so long that is it difficult to achieve clearance. These catheters are fine for more liquid material. Where the trachea requires direct suction, then the tracheal tube with an attached meconium aspirator may offer the best means of accessing this part of the airway (Figure 7.15).

Figure C7 Close up views of the ends of the three suction catheters shown in C.6 showing the difference in internal diameter as shown in the bottom picture, the Yankauer sucker (C) has a significantly greater internal diameter which combined with the shorter length makes it much more able to cope with thick particulate matter.

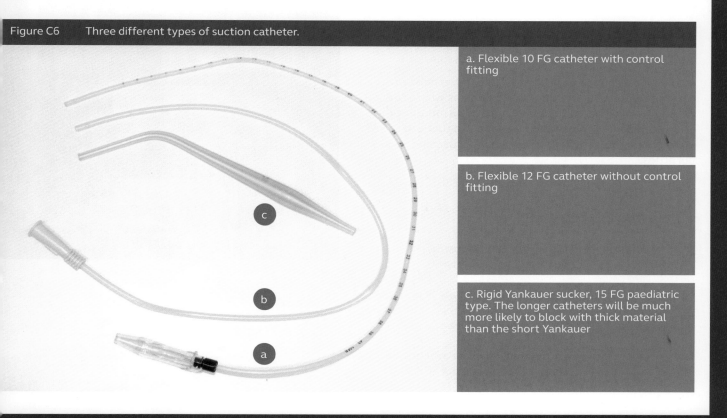

Figure C6   Three different types of suction catheter.

a. Flexible 10 FG catheter with control fitting

b. Flexible 12 FG catheter without control fitting

c. Rigid Yankauer sucker, 15 FG paediatric type. The longer catheters will be much more likely to block with thick material than the short Yankauer

Laryngoscopes

Laryngoscopes are useful if there is a need to inspect the airway and vital, should the need arise, to permit visualisation of the cords and trachea for intubation. There are differing types of laryngoscope and blade. The shape of the airway makes a straight bladed laryngoscope appropriate for neonatal use. Adult laryngoscopes have curved blades.

As a rule, longer blades can be used in smaller patients, but the opposite is not true, so it is difficult to visualise the cords in a large baby with a very short blade. Blades are described by their name and size. There are a number of different types of blade and it is a matter of individual preference as to which is felt to be the best. Much of the time there is no choice: you have to use what is available. If there is a choice then being able to recognise the different attributes can be helpful.

A variety of different types of laryngoscope blades are available and which are suitable for neonatal resuscitation. Typically a size 1 blade is used for larger term babies, a size 0 blade for smaller term babies and for most premature babies a size 00 blade might be required (Figure C8). The Seward and Miller blades are among the more commonly available and typified by a flat blade with a smaller, non-curving tongue-guard holding the tongue to the side. Wisconsin and Robertshaw blades (not shown) are similar. The Oxford blade (not shown) is characterised by a very large tongue guard curving over to create a tunnel through which it is possible to see the airway. This can be a challenge to insert in very small oral cavities but has the effect of holding the structures open.

Most new laryngoscopes have a high-intensity LED light source in the handle and a fibreoptic light guide in the blade. Blades may be re-useable or disposable.

Although unlikely to be routinely used in the newborn setting, there are also video laryngoscopes where the fibreoptic image from the blade is transmitted through to a video display. These can be useful in situations anticipating the 'difficult airway' and for teaching purposes.

Figure C7 — Close up views of the ends of the three suction catheters shown in C6 showing the difference in internal diameter as shown in the bottom picture, the Yankauer sucker (C) has a significantly greater internal diameter which combined with the shorter length makes it much more able to cope with thick particulate matter.

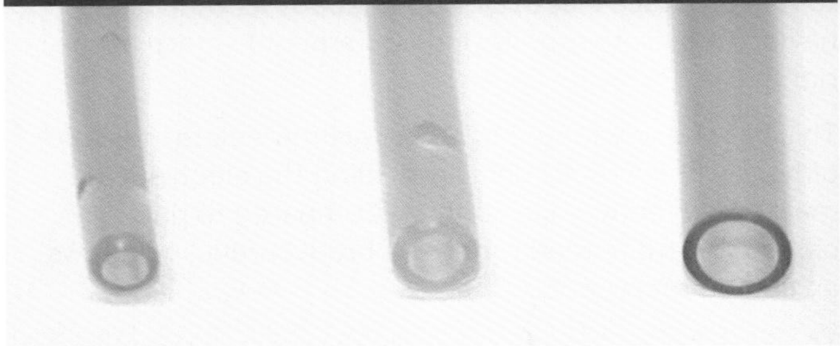

Figure C8 — Laryngoscope blades suitable for neonates and small infants.

The photograph shows (from top to bottom), a curved Macintosh paediatric blade (size 1), a straight Seward blade (size 1), a straight Miller blade (size 0) and a straight Miller blade (size 00). These are all fibre-optic blades with the handle containing the light source.

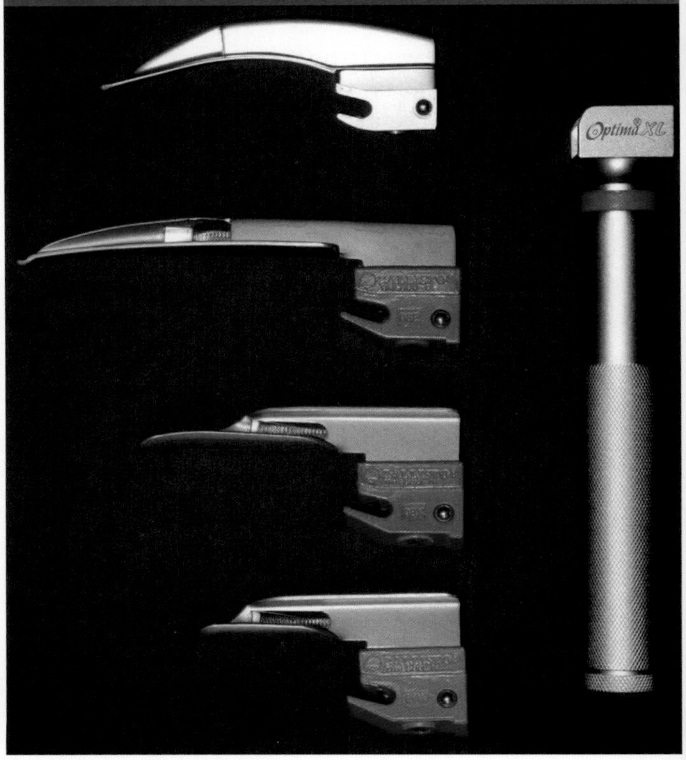

C: **Summary learning**

Equipment for the resuscitation of the newborn baby is continuously being developed and improved.

You should know how to check and operate the equipment available in your institution; this includes knowing what its advantages and disadvantages are.

You should also know what equipment is available, and how to use it, in the event of failure of your primary choice of equipment.

1. Wyckoff MH, Perlman JM, Laptook AR. Use of volume expansion during delivery room resuscitation in near-term and term infants. Pediatrics 2005;115:950–5.

2. Bjorland PA, Øymar K, Ersdal HL, Rettedal SI. Incidence of newborn resuscitative interventions at birth and short-term outcomes: a regional population-based study. BMJ Paediatr Open 2019;3:e000592.

3. Ersdal HL, Mduma E, Svensen E, Perlman JM. Early initiation of basic resuscitation interventions including face mask ventilation may reduce birth asphyxia related mortality in low-income countries: a prospective descriptive observational study. Resuscitation 2012;83:869–73.

4. Kc A, Lawn JE, Zhou H, et al. Not crying after birth as a predictor of not breathing. Pediatrics 2020;145:e20192719.

5. Morley CJ, Davis PG. Advances in neonatal resuscitation: supporting transition. Arch Dis Child Fetal Neonatal Ed 2008;93:F334–6.

6. Kroll L, Twohey L, Daubeney PE, et al. Risk factors at delivery and the need for skilled resuscitation. Eur J Obstet Gynecol Reprod Biol 1994;55:175–7.

7. Information & Statistics Division, Scottish Health Service. Hospital and Health Board Comparisons in Obstetrics 1988-90. 1992; 57.

8. Palme-Kilander C. Methods of resuscitation in low-Apgar-score in newborn infants – a national survey. Acta Paediatr 1992;81:739–44.

9. Allwood AC, Madar RJ, Baumer JH, et al. Changes in resuscitation practice at birth. Arch Dis Child Fetal Neonatal Ed 2003;88:F375–9.

10. Palme C, Nyström B, Tunell R. An evaluation of the efficiency of face masks in the resuscitation of newborn infants. Lancet 1985;1(8422):207–10.

11. Singh J, Santosh S, Wyllie JP, Mellon A. Effects of a course in neonatal resuscitation – evaluation of an educational intervention on the standard of neonatal resuscitation. Resuscitation 2006;68:385–9.

12. Perlman JM, Risser R. Cardiopulmonary resuscitation in the delivery room. Associated clinical events. Arch Pediatr Adolesc Med 1995;149:20–5.

13. Heathcote AC, Jones J, Clarke P. Timing and documentation of key events in neonatal resuscitation. Eur J Pediatr 2018;177:1053–6.

14. Primhak RA, Herber SM, Whincup G, Milner RDG. Which deliveries require paediatricians in attendance? Br Med J 1984;289:16–18.

15. van Henten TMA, Dekker J, Te Pas AB, et al. Tactile stimulation in the delivery room: do we practice what we preach? Arch Dis Child Fetal Neonatal Ed 2019;104:F661–2.

16. Dekker J, Martherus T, Cramer SJ, et al. Tactile stimulation to stimulate spontaneous breathing during stabilization of preterm infants at birth: A retrospective analysis. Front Pediatr 2017;5:61.

17. Baik-Schneditz N, Urlesberger B, Schwaberger B, et al. Tactile stimulation during neonatal transition and its effect on vital parameters in neonates during neonatal transition. Acta Paediatr 2018;107:952–7.

18. Wyckoff MH, Wyllie J, Aziz K, et al; Neonatal Life Support Collaborators. Neonatal Life Support 2020 International Consensus on Cardiopulmonary Resuscitation and Emergency Cardiovascular Care Science with Treatment Recommendations. Resuscitation 2020;156:A156–87.

19. Blank DA, Crossley KJ, Kashyap AJ, et al. Physiologic-based cord clamping maintains core temperature vs. immediate cord clamping in near-term lambs. Front Pediatr 2020;8:584983.

20. Bland RD. Lung liquid clearance before and after birth. Semin Perinatol 1988;12:124–33.

21. Lind J. Initiation of breathing in the newborn infant. J Ir Med Assoc 1962;50:88–93.

22. Walker D, Walker A, Wood C. Temperature of the human fetus. J Obstet Gynaecol Br Commonw 1969;76:503–11.

23. Currie AE. How cold can you get? A case of severe neonatal hypothermia. J R Soc Med 1994;87:293–4.

24. Dahm LS, James LS. Newborn temperature and calculated heat loss in the delivery room. Pediatrics 1972;49:504–13.

25. Stephenson JM, Du JN, Oliver TK. The effect of cooling on blood gas tensions in newborn infants. J Pediatr 1970;76:848–51.

26. Gandy GM, Adamsons K, Cunningham N, et al. Thermal environment and acid-base homeostasis in human infants during the first few hours of life. J Clin Invest 1964;43:751–8.

27. Gluck L, Kulovich MV, Eidelman AI, et al. Biochemical development of surface activity in mammalian lung. iv. Pulmonary lecithin synthesis in the human fetus and newborn and etiology of the respiratory distress syndrome. Pediatr Res 1972;6:81–99.

28. Macintosh M. (ed.). Project 27/28. An enquiry into quality of care and its effect on the survival of babies born at 27-28 weeks. Confidential Enquiry into Stillbirths and Deaths in Infancy. The Stationary Office, London, 2003.

29. Mullany LC, Katz J, Khatry SK, et al. Risk of mortality associated with neonatal hypothermia in southern Nepal. Arch Pediatr Adolesc Med 2010;164:650–6.

30. Wilson E, Maier RF, Norman M, et al; Effective Perinatal Intensive Care in Europe (EPICE) Research Group. Admission hypothermia in very preterm infants and neonatal mortality and morbidity. J Pediatr 2016;175:61–67.e4.

31. Madar J, Roehr CC, Ainsworth S, et al. European Resuscitation Council Guidelines 2021: Newborn resuscitation and support of transition of infants at birth. Resuscitation 2021;161:291–326.

32. Laptook AR, Salhab W, Bhaskar B; Neonatal Research Network. Admission temperature of low birth weight infants: predictors and associated morbidities. Pediatrics 2007;119:e643–9.

33. British Association of Perinatal Medicine. Therapeutic hypothermia for neonatal encephalopathy; a framework for practice. BAPM, London, 2020.

34. Johanson RB, Spencer SA, Rolfe P, et al. Effect of post-delivery care on neonatal body temperature. Acta Paediatr 1992;81:859–63.

35. Jia YS, Lin ZL, Lv H, et al. Effect of delivery room temperature on the admission temperature of premature infants: a randomized controlled trial. J Perinatol 2013;33:264–7.

36. Kent AL, Williams J. Increasing ambient operating theatre temperature and wrapping in polyethylene improves admission temperature in premature infants. J Paediatr Child Health 2008;44:325-31.

37. Nimbalkar SM, Patel VK, Patel DV, et al. Effect of early skin-to-skin contact following normal delivery on incidence of hypothermia in neonates more than 1800 g: randomized control trial. J Perinatol 2014;34:364–8.

38. Chamberlain R, Chamberlain G, Howlett B, Claireaux A. Chapter 4. The first breath. In: Chamberlain, R. British Births 1970. Volume 1: The first week of life. Heinemann Medical, London; 1975. p.89–117.

39. Owen CJ, Wyllie JP. Determination of heart rate in babies at birth. Resuscitation 2004;60:213–7.

40. Hawdon JM, Ward Platt MP, Aynsley-Green A. Patterns of metabolic adaptation for preterm and term infants in the first neonatal week. Arch Dis Child 1992;67:357–65.

41. Hawdon JM, Aynsley-Green A, Alberti KGMM, Ward Platt MP. The role of pancreatic insulin secretion in neonatal glucoregulation. 1. Healthy term and preterm infants. Arch Dis Child 1993;68:274–9.

42. Landon MB, Gabbe SG, Piana R, et al. Neonatal morbidity in pregnancy complicated by diabetes mellitus: predictive value of maternal glycemic profiles. Am J Obstet Gynecol 1987;156:1089–95.

43. Pruyn SC, Phelan JP, Buchanan GC. Long-term propranolol therapy in pregnancy: maternal and fetal outcome. Am J Obstet Gynecol 1979;135:485–9.

References

44. Becher JC, Bhushan SS, Lyon AJ. Unexpected collapse in apparently healthy newborns—a prospective national study of a missing cohort of neonatal deaths and near-death events. Arch Dis Child Fetal Neonatal Ed 2012;97:F30–4.

45. Monnelly V, Becher JC. Sudden unexpected postnatal collapse. Early Hum Dev 2018;126:28–31.

46. Andres V, Garcia P, Rimet Y, Nicaise C, Simeoni U. Apparent life-threatening events in presumably healthy newborns during early skin-to-skin contact. Pediatrics 2011;127:e1073–6.

47. Entwistle F. The evidence and rationale for the UNICEF UK baby friendly initiative standards. London: UNICEF; 2013.

48. Akerren Y, Furstenberg N. Gastrointestinal administration of oxygen in the treatment of asphyxia in the newborn. J Obstet Gynaecol Br Emp 1950;57:705–13.

49. Cooper EA, Smith H, Pask EA. On the efficiency of intragastric oxygen. Anaesthesia 1960;15:211–28.

50. Coxon RV. The effect of intragastric oxygen on the oxygenation of arterial and portal blood in hypoxic animals. Lancet 1960;i:1315–7.

51. Barrie H, Cottom DG, Wilson BDR. Respiratory stimulants in the newborn. Lancet 1962;ii:742–6.

52. Daniel SS, Dawes GS, James LS, Ross BB. Analeptics and resuscitation of asphyxiated monkeys. Br Med J 1966;ii:562–3.

53. Godfrey S. Blood gases during asphyxia and resuscitation of fetal and newborn rabbits. Respir Physiol 1968;4:309–21.

54. Eve FC. Actuation of the inert diaphragm by a gravity method. Lancet 1932;ii:995–7.

55. Eve FC. Complacency in resuscitation of the drowned. Br Med J 1943;i:535–7.

56. Handley DB, Handley D. A rocker for asphyxia neonatorum. Br Med J 1951;ii:1282.

57. Cross KW, Dawes GS, Hyman A, Mott JC. Hyperbaric oxygen and intermittent positive pressure ventilation in resuscitation of asphyxiated newborn rabbits. Lancet 1964;ii:560–2.

58. Hutchison J, Kerr M, Williams K, Hopkinson W. Hyperbaric oxygen in the resuscitation of the newborn. Lancet 1963;ii:1019–22.

59. Cordey R, Chiolero R, Miller J Jr. Resuscitation of neonates by hypothermia: report of 20 cases with acid-base determination on 10 cases and longterm development of 33 cases. Resuscitation 1973;2:169–87.

60. Westin B, Miller J, Nyberg R, Wedenberg E. Neonatal asphyxia pallida treated with hypothermia alone or with hypothermia and transfusion of oxygenated blood. Surgery 1959;45:868–79.

61. Edwards AD, Brocklehurst P, Gunn AJ, et al. Neurological outcomes at 18 months of age after moderate hypothermia for perinatal hypoxic ischaemic encephalopathy: synthesis and meta-analysis of trial data. Brit Med J 2010;340:363c.

62. Dawes G. Chapter 12. Birth Asphyxia, Resuscitation and Brain Damage. In: Foetal and neonatal physiology. Year Book Publisher, Chicago, 1968. p.141–59.

63. Cross KW. Resuscitation of the asphyxiated infant. Brit Med Bull 1966;22:73–8.

64. Godfrey S. Respiratory and cardiovascular changes during asphyxia and resuscitation of foetal newborn rabbits. Q J Exp Physiol Cogn Med Sci 1968;53:97–118.

65. van Vonderen JJ, Roest AA, Siew ML, et al. Measuring physiological changes during the transition to life after birth. Neonatology 2014;105:230–42.

66. Siew ML, Wallace MJ, Kitchen MJ, et al. Inspiration regulates the rate and temporal pattern of lung liquid clearance and lung aeration at birth. J Appl Physiol (1985) 2009;106:1888–95.

67. Blank DA, Kamlin COF, Rogerson SR, et al. Lung ultrasound during the initiation of breathing in healthy term and late preterm infants immediately after birth, a prospective, observational study. Resuscitation 2017;114:59–65.

68. Hooper SB, Crossley KJ, Zahra VA, et al. Effect of body position and ventilation on umbilical artery and venous blood flows during delayed umbilical cord clamping in preterm lambs. Arch Dis Child Fetal Neonatal Ed 2017;102:F312–9.

69. Hooper SB, te Pas AB, Lang J, et al. Cardiovascular transition at birth: a physiological sequence. Pediatr Res 2015;77:608–14.

70. Safar P, Escarraga LA, Elam JO. A comparison of the mouth-to-mouth and mouth-to-airway methods of artificial respiration with chest-pressure arm-lift methods. N Engl J Med 1958;258:671–7.

71. Kouwenhoven WB, Jude JR, Knickerbocker GG. Closed-chest cardiac massage. JAMA 1960;173:1064–7.

72. Moya F, James LS, Bernard E, Hanks EC. Closed chest cardiac massage in the newborn. Anaesthesiol 1961;22:644–5.

73. Hamer Hodges RJ, Tunstall ME, Knight RF, Wilson EJ. Endotracheal aspiration and oxygenation in resuscitation of the newborn. Br J Anaesth 1960;32:9–15.

74. Tunstall ME, Hodges RJH. A sterile disposable neonatal tracheal tube. Lancet 1961;i:146.

75. Flagg PJ. The treatment of asphyxia in the newborn. JAMA 1928;91:788–91.

76. Hooper SB, te Pas AB, Lewis RA, Morley CJ. Establishing functional residual capacity at birth. NeoReviews 2010;11: e474–83.

77. te Pas AB, Davis PG, Hooper SB, Morley CJ. From liquid to air: breathing after birth. J Pediatr 2008;152:607–11.

78. Hooper SB, Harding R. Fetal lung liquid: a major determinant of the growth and functional development of the fetal lung. Clin Exp Pharmacol Physiol 1995;22:235–47.

79. Harding R, Hooper SB. Regulation of lung expansion and lung growth before birth. J Appl Physiol (1985) 1996;81:209–24.

80. Prsa M, Sun L, van Amerom J, et al. Reference ranges of blood flow in the major vessels of the normal human fetal circulation at term by phase-contrast magnetic resonance imaging. Circ Cardiovasc Imaging 2014;7:663–70.

81. Rudolph AM, Heymann MA, Teramo KAW, Barrett CT, Räihä NCR. Studies on the circulation of the previable human fetus. Pediatr Res 1971;5:452–65.

82. Kiserud T, Rasmussen S, Sethi V. Fetal blood flow distribution to the placenta. Ultrasound Obstet Gynecol 2003;22 (suppl S1):37.

83. Walters DW, Olver RE. The role of catecholamines in lung liquid absorption at birth. Pediatr Res 1978;12:239–42.

84. Strang LB. Fetal lung liquid: secretion and reabsorption. Physiol Rev 1991;71:991–1016.

85. Berger PJ, Kyriakides MA, Smolich JJ, Ramsden CA, Walker AM. Massive decline in lung liquid before vaginal delivery at term in the fetal lamb. Am J Obstet Gynecol 1998;178:223–7.

86. Olver RE, Ramsden CA, Strang LB, Walters DV. The role of amiloride blockable sodium transport in adrenaline-induced lung liquid reabsorption in the fetal lamb. J Physiol 1986;376:321–40.

87. Caravagna C, Seaborn T. Oxygen sensing in early life. Lung 2016;194:715–22.

88. Thorburn GD. The placenta and the control of fetal breathing movements. Reprod Fertil Dev 1995;7:577–94.

89. Watson CS, Homan JH, White SE, Challis JR, Bocking AD. Prostaglandin E2 inhibition of fetal breathing movements is not sustained during prolonged reduced uterine blood flow in sheep. Can J Physiol Pharmacol 1998;76:858–66.

90. Soothill PW, Nicolaides KH, Rodeck CH, Gamsu H. Blood gases and acid-base status of the human second-trimester fetus. Obstet Gynecol 1986;68:173–6.

91. Stuart B, Drumm J, FitzGerald DE, Duignan NM. Fetal blood velocity waveforms in uncomplicated labour. Br J Obstet Gynaecol 1981;88:865–9.

92. Peebles DM, Edwards AD, Wyatt JS, et al. Changes in human fetal cerebral oxygenation and blood volume during delivery. Am J Obstet Gynecol 1992;167:1916–7.

93. Adamson SL, Richardson BS, Homan J. Initiation of pulmonary gas exchange by fetal sheep in utero. J Appl Physiol (1985) 1987;62:989–98.

94. Adamson SL, Kuipers IM, Olson DM. Umbilical cord occlusion stimulates breathing independent of blood gases and pH. J Appl Physiol (1985) 1991;70:1796–809.

95. Hooper SB, Siew ML, Kitchen MJ, te Pas AB. Establishing functional residual capacity in the non-breathing infant. Semin Fetal Neonatal Med 2013;18:336–43.

96. Condorelli S, Scarpelli EM. Somatic-respiratory reflex and onset of regular breathing movements in the lamb fetus in utero. Pediatr Res 1975;9:879–84.

97. Bland RD. Loss of liquid from the lung lumen in labor: More than a simple 'squeeze'. Am J Physiol Lung Cell Mol Physiol 2001;280: L602–5.

98. Hooper SB, Te Pas AB, Kitchen MJ. Respiratory transition in the newborn: a three-phase process. Arch Dis Child Fetal Neonatal Ed 2016;101:F266–71.

99. Hooper SB, Kitchen MJ, Siew ML, et al. Imaging lung aeration and lung liquid clearance at birth using phase contrast X-ray imaging. Clin Exp Pharmacol Physiol 2009;36:117–25.

100. Vyas H, Milner AD, Hopkin IE. Intra-thoracic pressure and volume changes during the spontaneous onset of respiration in babies born by cesarean-section and by vaginal delivery. J Pediatr 1981;99:787–91.

101. Hooper SB, Kitchen MJ, Wallace MJ, et al. Imaging lung aeration and lung liquid clearance at birth. FASEB J 2007;21:3329–37.

102. Miserocchi G, Poskurica BH, Del Fabbro M. Pulmonary interstitial pressure in anesthetized paralyzed newborn rabbits. J Appl Physiol 1994;77:2260–8.

103. te Pas AB, Siew M, Wallace MJ, et al. Establishing functional residual capacity at birth: the effect of sustained inflation and positive end expiratory pressure in a preterm rabbit model. Pediatr Res 2009;65:537–41.

104. Blank DA, Gaertner VD, Kamlin COF, et al. Respiratory changes in term infants immediately after birth. Resuscitation 2018;130:105–10.

105. Gao Y, Raj JU. Regulation of the pulmonary circulation in the fetus and newborn. Physiol Rev 2010;90:1291–335.

106. Bhatt S, Alison BJ, Wallace EM, et al. Delaying cord clamping until ventilation onset improves cardiovascular function at birth in preterm lambs. J Physiol 2013;591:2113–26.

107. Crossley KJ, Allison BJ, Polglase GR, et al. Dynamic changes in the direction of blood flow through the ductus arteriosus at birth. J Physiol 2009;587:4695–704.

108. Dawson JA, Kamlin CO, Wong C, et al. Changes in heart rate in the first minutes after birth. Arch Dis Child Fetal Neonatal Ed 2010;95:F177–81.

109. Brady JP, James LS. Heart rate changes in the fetus and newborn infant during labor, delivery, and the immediate neonatal period. Am J Obstet Gynecol 1962;84:1–12.

110. Oh W, Lind J, Gessner IH. The circulatory and respiratory adaptation to early and late cord clamping in newborn infants. Acta Paediatr Scand 1966;55:17–25.

111. Lind J, Peltonen T, Tornwall L, Wegelius C. Roentgenological lung findings in the newborn infant's 1st breath. Z Kinderheilkd 1963;87:568–78.

112. Arcilla RA, Lind J. Serial phonocardiography during the neonatal period. A comparative study in infants born with early and late clamping of the cord. Z Kinderheilkd 1965;93:354–74.

113. Peltonen T. Placental transfusion – advantage and disadvantage. Eur J Pediatr 1981;137:141–6.

114. van Vonderen JJ, Roest AAW, Klumper FJC, Hooper SB, Te Pas AB. The effect of breathing on ductus arteriosus blood flow directly after birth. Eur J Pediatr 2017;176:1581–5.

115. Blank DA, Badurdeen S, Kamlin COF, et al. Baby-directed umbilical cord clamping: A feasibility study. Resuscitation 2018;131:1–7.

116. Farrar D, Airey R, Law GR, Tuffnell D, Cattle B, Duley L. Measuring placental transfusion for term births: weighing babies with cord intact. BJOG 2011;118:70–5.

117. Vandenberghe G, Bloemenkamp K, Berlage S, et al; INOSS (the International Network of Obstetric Survey Systems). The International Network of Obstetric Survey Systems study of uterine rupture: a descriptive multi-country population-based study. BJOG 2019;126:370–81.

118. Downes KL, Grantz KL, Shenassa ED. Maternal, Labor, Delivery, and Perinatal Outcomes Associated with Placental Abruption: A Systematic Review. Am J Perinatol 2017;34:935–57.

119. Murphy DJ, MacKenzie IZ. The mortality and morbidity associated with umbilical cord prolapse. Br J Obstet Gynaecol 1995;102:826–30.

120. Mercer J, Erickson-Owens D, Skovgaard R. Cardiac asystole at birth: Is hypovolemic shock the cause? Med Hypotheses 2009;72:458–63.

121. Nasiell J, Papadogiannakis N, Löf E, Elofsson F, Hallberg B. Hypoxic ischemic encephalopathy in newborns linked to placental and umbilical cord abnormalities. J Matern Fetal Neonatal Med 2016;29:721–6.

122. Moore WMO, Davis JA. Response of the newborn rabbit to acute anoxia and variations due to narcotic agents. Br J Anaesth 1966;38:787–92.

123. Hey E, Kelly J. Gaseous exchange during endotracheal ventilation for asphyxia at birth. J Obstet Gynaecol Br Commonw 1968;75: 414–24.

124. Ditchburn RK, Hull D, Segall MM. Oxygen uptake during and after positive-pressure ventilation for the resuscitation of asphyxiated newborn infants. Lancet 1966;ii:1096–9.

125. Avila-Alvarez A, Davis PG, Kamlin COF, Thio M. Documentation during neonatal resuscitation: a systematic review. Arch Dis Child Fetal Neonatal Ed 2020 Nov 26:fetalneonatal-2020-319948. [Epub ahead of print].

126. Dekker J, Hooper SB, Martherus T, et al. Repetitive versus standard tactile stimulation of preterm infants at birth - A randomized controlled trial. Resuscitation 2018;127:37–43.

127. O'Donnell CPF, Kamlin COF, Davis PG, et al. Clinical assessment of infant colour at delivery. Arch Dis Child Fetal Neonatal Ed 2007;92:F465–7.

128. Smit M, Dawson JA, Ganzeboom A, et al. Pulse oximetry in newborns with delayed cord clamping and immediate skin-to-skin contact. Arch Dis Child Fetal Neonatal Ed 2014;99:F309–14.

129. Katheria A, Rich W, Finer N. Electrocardiogram provides a continuous heart rate faster than oximetry during neonatal resuscitation. Pediatrics 2012;130:e1177–81.

130. Luong D, Cheung PY, Barrington KJ, et al. Cardiac arrest with pulseless electrical activity rhythm in newborn infants: a case series. Arch Dis Child Fetal Neonatal Ed 2019;104:F572–4.

131. Louis D, Sundaram V, Kumar P. Pulse oximeter sensor application during neonatal resuscitation: a randomized controlled trial. Pediatrics 2014;133:476–82.

132. Pinnamaneni R, Kieran EA, O'Donnell CP. Speed of data display by pulse oximeters in newborns: a randomised crossover study. Arch Dis Child Fetal Neonatal Ed 2010;95:F384–5.

133. O'Donnell CP, Kamlin CO, Davis PG, Morley CJ. Feasibility of and delay in obtaining pulse oximetry during neonatal resuscitation. J Pediatr 2005;147:698–9.

134. Dawson JA, Kamlin CO, Vento M, et al. Defining the reference range for oxygen saturation for infants after birth. Pediatrics 2010;125:e1340–7.

135. Falciglia HS, Henderschott C, Potter P, Helmchen R. Does De Lee suction at the perineum prevent meconium aspiration syndrome. Am J Obstet Gynecol 1992;167:1243–9.

136. Trevisanuto D, Strand ML, Kawakami MD, et al; International Liaison Committee on Resuscitation Neonatal Life Support Task Force. Tracheal suctioning of meconium at birth for non-vigorous infants: a systematic review and meta-analysis. Resuscitation 2020;149:117–26.

References

137. Hull D. Lung expansion and ventilation during resuscitation of asphyxiated newborn infants. J Pediatr 1969;75:47–58.

138. Vyas H, Milner AD, Hopkin IE, Boon AW. Physiologic responses to prolonged and slow rise inflation in the resuscitation of the asphyxiated newborn infant. J Pediatr 1981;99:635–9.

139. Lamberska T, Luksova M, Smisek J, et al. Premature infants born at <25 weeks of gestation may be compromised by currently recommended resuscitation techniques. Acta Paediatr 2016;105:e142-50.

140. Bhat P, Hunt K, Harris C, et al. Inflation pressures and times during initial resuscitation in preterm infants. Pediatr Int 2017;59:906–10.

141. Eilevstjønn J, Linde JE, Blacy L, Kidanto H, Ersdal HL. Distribution of heart rate and responses to rescitation among 1237 apnoeic newborns at birth. Resuscitation 2020;152:69–76.

142. Marlow N, Bennett C, Draper ES, et al. Perinatal outcomes for extremely preterm babies in relation to place of birth in England: the EPICure 2 study. Arch Dis Child Fetal Neonatal Ed 2014;99:F181-8.

143. Gale C, Santhakumaran S, Nagarajan S, et al; Neonatal Data Analysis Unit and the Medicines for Neonates Investigator Group. Impact of managed clinical networks on NHS specialist neonatal services in England: population based study. BMJ 2012;344:e2105.

144. British Association of Perinatal Medicine. Perinatal management of extreme preterm birth before 27 weeks of gestation. A framework for practice. BAPM, London, 2019.

145. Mellander M. Perinatal management, counselling and outcome of fetuses with congenital heart disease. Semin Fetal Neonatal Med 2005;10:586-93.

146. Berazategui JP, Aguilar A, Escobedo M, et al; ANR study group. Risk factors for advanced resuscitation in term and near-term infants: a case-control study. Arch Dis Child Fetal Neonatal Ed 2017;102:F44-F50.

147. Aziz K, Chadwick M, Baker M, Andrews W. Ante- and intra-partum factors that predict increased need for neonatal resuscitation. Resuscitation 2008;79:444-52.

148. Russ S, Rout S, Sevdalis N, Moorthy K, Darzi A, Vincent C. Do safety checklists improve teamwork and communication in the operating room? A systematic review. Ann Surg 2013;258:856–71.

149. Sewell RD, Steinberg MA. Chest compressions in an infant with osteogenesis imperfecta type II: no new rib fractures. Pediatrics 2000;106:e71.

150. Scott RJ, Goodburn SF. Potter's syndrome in the second trimester— prenatal screening and pathological findings in 60 cases of oligohydramnios sequence. Prenat Diagn 1995;15:519–25.

151. Kirkup B. The Report of The Morecambe Bay Investigation. The Stationery Office, London, 2015. (available at https://www.gov.uk/government/publications/morecambe-bay-investigation-report - accessed 21 January 2021)

152. Royal College of Obstetricians and Gynaecologists. Each Baby Counts: 2015 full report. London: RCOG; 2017.

153. Draper ES, Gallimore ID, Smith LK, et al, on behalf of the MBRRACE-UK Collaboration. MBRRACE-UK Perinatal Mortality Surveillance Report, UK Perinatal Deaths for Births from January to December 2017. Leicester: The Infant Mortality and Morbidity Studies, Department of Health Sciences, University of Leicester. 2019.

154. Ockenden D. Emerging Findings and Recommendations from the Independent Review of Maternity Services at the Shrewsbury and Telford Hospital NHS Trust. The Stationery Office, London, 2020. (available at https://www.ockendenmaternityreview.org.uk/wp-content/uploads/2020/12/ockenden-report.pdf - accessed 21 January 2021)

155. National Institute for Health and Care Excellence (NICE). Intrapartum care: care of healthy women and their babies during childbirth. Clinical Guideline 190 (CG190). National Institute for Health and Care Excellence. London, 2014. (updated 2017).

156. Janvier A, Barrington K, Farlow B. Communication with parents concerning withholding or withdrawing of life-sustaining interventions in neonatology. Semin Perinatol 2014;38:38–46.

157. Inch S. Management of the third stage of labour – a cascade of intervention? Midwifery 1985;1:114–22

158. Dunn PM. Aristotle (384–322 BC): philosopher and scientist of ancient Greece. Arch Dis Child Fetal Neonatal Ed 2006;91:F75–7.

159. White, C. A treatise on the management of pregnant and lying-in women. London: Edward and Charles Dilly, 1773.

160. McClintock AH, ed. Smellie's treatise on the theory and practice of midwifery. Vols I, II, & III. London: The New Sydenham Society, 1876-78.

161. Magennis E. A Midwifery surgical clamp. Lancet 1899;153:1373.

162. Goodall JR, Andersen FO, Altimas GT, MacPhail FL. An inexhaustible source of blood for transfusion and its preservation. Surg Gynecol Obstet 1938;66:176-8.

163. Grodberg BC, Carey EL. A study of seventy-five transfusions with placental blood. N Engl J Med 1938;219:471–4.

164. Rogers J, Wood J, McCandlish R, et al. Active versus expectant management of the third stage of labour: the Hinchingbrooke randomised controlled trial. Lancet 1998;351:693–99.

165. Parliamentary Office of Science and Technology Caesarean Sections. 2002. Available on the worldwide web at http://www.parliament.uk/documents/post/pn184.pdf - accessed 21 November 2020)

166. Jelin AC, Kuppermann M, Erickson K, Clyman R, Schulkin J. Obstetricians' attitudes and beliefs regarding umbilical cord clamping. J Matern Fetal Neonatal Med 2014;27:1457–61.

167. Sawyer A, Ayers S, Bertullies S, et al. Providing immediate neonatal care and resuscitation at birth beside the mother: parents' views, a qualitative study. BMJ Open 2015;5:e008495.

168. Guttmann K, Martin A, Chaudhary A, Cole J, Foglia EE. Resuscitation before cord clamping: the maternal experience. Arch Dis Child Fetal Neonatal Ed 2020;105:569-570.

169. Gomersall J, Berber S, Middleton P, et al; on behalf of the International Liaison Committee on Resuscitation. Umbilical Cord Management at Term and Late Preterm Birth: A Systematic Review and Meta-Analysis. Pediatrics 2021;147:e2020015404.

170. Seidler AL, Gyte GML, Rabe H, et al; International Liaison Committee on Resuscitation Neonatal Life Support Task Force. Umbilical Cord Management for Newborns <34 Weeks' Gestation: A Meta-analysis. Pediatrics 2021;147:e20200576.

171. Batey N, Yoxall CW, Fawke JA, Duley L, Dorling J. Fifteen-minute consultation: stabilisation of the high-risk newborn infant beside the mother. Arch Dis Child Educ Pract Ed 2017;102:235-238.

172. Katheria AC, Brown MK, Faksh A, et al. Delayed cord clamping in newborns born at term at risk for resuscitation: a feasibility randomized clinical trial. J Pediatr 2017;187:313–7.e1.

173. Polglase GR, Blank DA, Barton SK, et al. Physiologically based cord clamping stabilises cardiac output and reduces cerebrovascular injury in asphyxiated near-term lambs. Arch Dis Child Fetal Neonatal Ed 2018;103:F530–8.

174. Andersson O, Rana N, Ewald U, et al. Intact cord resuscitation versus early cord clamping in the treatment of depressed newborn infants during the first 10 minutes of birth (Nepcord III) - a randomized clinical trial. Matern Health Neonatol Perinatol 2019;5:15.

175. McAdams RM, Fay E, Delaney S. Whole blood volumes associated with milking intact and cut umbilical cords in term newborns. J Perinatol 2018;38:245–50.

176. Katheria AC, Truong G, Cousins L, Oshiro B, Finer NN. Umbilical cord milking versus delayed cord clamping in preterm infants. Pediatrics 2015;136:61–9.

177. Upadhyay A, Gothwal S, Parihar R, et al. Effect of umbilical cord milking in term and near term infants: randomized control trial. Am J Obstet Gynecol 2013;208:120.e1–6.

178. Katheria A, Reister F, Essers J, et al. Association of umbilical cord milking vs delayed umbilical cord clamping with death or severe intraventricular hemorrhage among preterm infants. JAMA 2019;322:1877-1886.

179. Blank DA, Polglase GR, Kluckow M, et al. Haemodynamic effects of umbilical cord milking in premature sheep during the neonatal transition. Arch Dis Child Fetal Neonatal Ed 2018;103:F539-F546.

180. Stephens RH, Benjamin AR, Walters DV. Volume and protein concentration of epithelial lining liquid in perfused in situ postnatal sheep lungs. Am J Physiol 1996;80:1911–20.

181. Ramachandrappa A, Jain L. Elective cesarean section: its impact on neonatal respiratory outcome. Clin Perinatol 2008;35:373–93.

182. Milner AD, Saunders RA. Pressure and volume changes in the first breath of human neonates. Arch Dis Child 1977;52:918–24.

183. Boon AW, Milner AD, Hopkin IE. Physiological responses of the newborn infant to resuscitation. Arch Dis Child 1979;54:492–8.

184. Kapadia VS, Urlesberger B, Soraisham A, et al; International Liaison Committee on Resuscitation Neonatal Life Support Task Force. Sustained Lung Inflations During Neonatal Resuscitation at Birth: A Meta-analysis. Pediatrics 2021;147:e2020021204.

185. Kirpalani H, Ratcliffe SJ, Keszler M, et al; SAIL Site Investigators. Effect of sustained inflations vs intermittent positive pressure ventilation on bronchopulmonary dysplasia or death among extremely preterm infants: The SAIL randomized clinical trial. JAMA 2019;321:1165–75.

186. Morley CJ, Dawson JA, Stewart MJ, et al. The effect of a PEEP valve on a Laerdal neonatal self-inflating resuscitation bag. J Paediatr Child Health 2010;46:51–6.

187. Finer NN, Rich W, Craft A, Henderson C. Comparison of methods of bag and mask ventilation for neonatal resuscitation. Resuscitation 2001;49:299–305.

188. Bennett S, Finer NN, Rich W, Vaucher Y. A comparison of three neonatal resuscitation devices. Resuscitation 2005;67:113–8.

189. Wood FE, Morley CJ. Face mask ventilation – the dos and don'ts. Semin Fetal Neonatal Med 2013;18:344–51.

190. Wood FE, Platten CR, Byrne S, Wyllie JP. Manikin based studies of simulated resuscitation practices: Term Face Mask Study. Pediatr Res 2011;70:752 (abstract).

191. Wood FE, Platten CR, Byrne S, Wyllie JP. Manikin based studies of simulated resuscitation practices: Preterm Face Mask Study. Pediatr Res 2011;70:104 (abstract).

192. Wood FE, Morley CJ, Dawson JA, et al. Assessing the effectiveness of two round neonatal resuscitation masks: study 1. Arch Dis Child Fetal Neonatal Ed 2008;93:F235–7.

193. O'Shea JE, Thio M, Owen LS, et al. Measurements from preterm infants to guide face mask size. Measurements from preterm infants to guide face mask size. Arch Dis Child Fetal Neonatal Ed 2016;101: F294–8.

194. Haase B, Badinska AM, Koos B, et al. Do commonly available round facemasks fit near-term and term infants? Arch Dis Child Fetal Neonatal Ed 2020;105:F364–8.

195. Wood FE, Morley CJ, Dawson JA, et al. Improved techniques reduce face mask leak during simulated neonatal resuscitation: study 2. Arch Dis Child Fetal Neonatal Ed 2008;93:F230–4.

196. Yam CH, Dawson JA, Schmölzer GM, et al. Heart rate changes during resuscitation of newly born infants <30 weeks gestation: an observational study. Arch Dis Child Fetal Neonatal Ed 2011;96:F102–7.

197. Tracy MB, Klimek J, Coughtrey H, et al. Mask leak in one-person mask ventilation compared to two-person in a newborn infant manikin study. Arch Dis Child Fetal Neonatal Ed 2011;96:F195–200.

198. Bansal SC, Caoci S, Dempsey E, et al. The laryngeal mask airway and its use in neonatal resuscitation: A critical review of where we are in 2017/2018. Neonatology 2018;113:152–61.

199. Fernández-Jurado MI, Fernández-Baena M. Use of laryngeal mask airway for prolonged ventilatory support in a preterm newborn. Paediatr Anaesth 2002;12:369–70.

200. Trevisanuto D, Parotto M, Doglioni N, et al. Upper esophageal lesion following laryngeal mask airway resuscitation in a very low birth weight infant. Resuscitation 2011;82:1251–2.

201. Pejovic NJ, Myrnerts Höök S, Byamugisha J, et al. A randomized trial of laryngeal mask airway in neonatal resuscitation. N Engl J Med 2020;383:2138–47.

202. Pejovic NJ, Trevisanuto D, Lubulwa C, et al. Neonatal resuscitation using a laryngeal mask airway: a randomised trial in Uganda. Arch Dis Child 2018;103:255–60.

203. Gandini D, Brimacombe J. Manikin training for neonatal resuscitation with the laryngeal mask airway. Paediatr Anaesth 2004;14:493–4.

204. Galderisi A, De Bernardo G, Lorenzon E, Trevisanuto D. iGel: a new supraglottic device for effective resuscitation of a very low birthweight infant with Cornelia de Lange syndrome. BMJ Case Rep 2015 Mar 25;2015.

205. Kamlin COF, Schmölzer GM, Dawson JA, et al. A randomized trial of oropharyngeal airways to assist stabilization of preterm infants in the delivery room. Resuscitation 2019;144:106–14.

206. Wiswell TE, Tuggle JM, Turner BS. Meconium aspiration syndrome: have we made a difference? Pediatrics 1990;85:715–21.

207. Dillard RG. Neonatal tracheal aspiration of meconium-stained infants. J Pediatr 1977;90:163–4.

208. Chettri S, Adhisivam B, Bhat BV. Endotracheal suction for nonvigorous neonates born through meconium stained amniotic fluid: a randomized controlled trial. J Pediatr 2015;166:1208–13. e1.

209. Nangia S, Sunder S, Biswas R, Saili A. Endotracheal suction in term non vigorous meconium stained neonates-a pilot study. Resuscitation 2016;105:79–84.

210. Singh SN, Saxena S, Bhriguvanshi A, et al. Effect of endotracheal suctioning just after birth in non-vigorous infants born through meconium stained amniotic fluid: a randomized controlled trial. Clin Epidemiol Glob Health 2019;7:165–70.

211. Vain NE, Szyld EG, Prudent LM, et al. Oropharyngeal and nasopharyngeal suctioning of meconium-stained neonates before delivery of their shoulders: multicentre, randomised controlled trial. Lancet 2004:364;597–602.

212. Wiswell TE, Gannon CM, Jacob J, et al. Delivery room management of the apparently vigorous meconium-stained neonate: results of the multicenter, international collaborative trial. Pediatrics 2000;105:1–7.

213. Oei JL, Finer NN, Saugstad OD, et al. Outcomes of oxygen saturation targeting during delivery room stabilisation of preterm infants. Arch Dis Child Fetal Neonatal Ed 2018;103:F446–54.

214. Thió M, Bhatia R, Dawson JA, Davis PG. Oxygen delivery using neonatal self-inflating resuscitation bags without a reservoir. Arch Dis Child Fetal Neonatal Ed 2010;95:F315–9.

215. Reise K, Monkman S, Kirpalani H. The use of the Laerdal infant resuscitator results in the delivery of high oxygen fractions in the absence of a blender. Resuscitation 2009;80:120–5.

216. Finer NN, Barrington KJ, Al-Fadley F, et al. Limitations of self-inflating resuscitators. Pediatrics 1986;77:417–20.

217. Boon AW, Milner AD, Hopkin IE. Lung expansion, tidal exchange, and formation of the functional residual capacity during resuscitation of asphyxiated neonates. J Pediatr 1979;95:1031–6.

218. Martherus T, Oberthuer A, Dekker J, et al. Supporting breathing of preterm infants at birth: a narrative review. Arch Dis Child Fetal Neonatal Ed 2019;104:F102–7.

219. Poets CF, Rüdiger M. Mask CPAP during neonatal transition: too much of a good thing for some term infants? Arch Dis Child Fetal Neonatal Ed 2015;100:F378–9.

220. Claassen CC, Strand ML. Understanding the risks and benefits of delivery room CPAP for term infants. Pediatrics 2019;144:e20191720.

221. Hishikawa K, Goishi K, Fujiwara T, et al. Pulmonary air leak associated with CPAP at term birth resuscitation. Arch Dis Child Fetal Neonatal Ed 2015;100:F382–7.

222. Clevenger L, Britton JR. Delivery room continuous positive airway pressure and early pneumothorax in term newborn infants. J Neonatal Perinatal Med 2017;10:157–61.

References

223. Smithhart W, Wyckoff MH, Kapadia V, et al. Delivery room continuous positive airway pressure and pneumothorax. Pediatrics 2019;144:e20190756.

224. Tonkin SL, Davis SL, Gunn TR. Nasal route for infant resuscitation by mothers. Lancet 1995;345:1353–4.

225. Niles DE, Cines C, Insley E, et al. Incidence and characteristics of positive pressure ventilation delivered to newborns in a US tertiary academic hospital. Resuscitation 2017;115:102–9.

226. Barber CA, Wyckoff MH. Use and efficacy of endotracheal versus intravenous epinephrine during neonatal cardiopulmonary resuscitation in the delivery room. Pediatrics 2006;118:1028–34.

227. Huynh T, Hemway RJ, Perlman JM. Assessment of effective face mask ventilation is compromised during synchronised chest compressions. Arch Dis Child Fetal Neonatal Ed 2015;100:F39–42.

228. Hake TG. Studies on ether and chloroform from Professor Schiff's physiological laboratory. Practitioner 1874;12: 241.

229. Schiff M. Ueber direkte reizung der herzoberflaeche. Arch Ges Physiol 1882;28:200.

230. Boehm R. Ueber wiederbelebung nach vergiftungen und asphyxia. Arch Exp Pathol Pharm 1878;8:68.

231. Maass F. Die methode der wiederbelebung bei herztod nach chloroformeinathmung. Berlin Klin Wochenschr 1892;29:265–8.

232. Galos G, Surks S. Cardiorespiratory arrest in the newborn treated by cardiac massage. Am J Obstet Gynecol 1957;74:1108–11.

233. Reilly RJ, Melville HA. Cardiac massage in the resuscitation of a stillborn infant. Br Med J 1962;i:91–2.

234. Halperin M. Heart massage in a newborn infant. JAMA 1957;164:1996.

235. Sutherland JM, Epple HH. Cardiac massage of stillborn infants. Obstet Gynecol 1961;18:182–6.

236. Gallagher B, Neligan G. Resuscitation of the stillborn infant. Br Med J 1962;i:400.

237. Thaler MM, Stobie GHC. An improved technic of external cardiac compression in infants and young children. N Engl J Med 1963;269:606–10.

238. Rudikoff MT, Maughan WL, Effron M, et al. Mechanisms of blood flow during cardiopulmonary resuscitation. Circulation 1980;61:345–52.

239. Del Guercio LRM, Coomaraswamy RP, State D. Cardiac output and other hemodynamic variables during external cardiac massage in man. N Engl J Med 1963;269:1398–404.

240. Voorhees WD, Babbs CF, Tacker WA. Regional blood flow during cardiopulmonary resuscitation in dogs. Crit Care Med 1980;8:134–6.

241. Berg RA, Sanders AB, Kern KB, et al. Adverse effects of interrupting chest compressions for rescue breathing during cardiopulmonary resuscitation for ventricular fibrillation cardiac arrest. Circulation 2001;104:2465–70.

242. Todres ID, Rogers MC. Methods of external cardiac massage in the newborn infant. J Pediatr 1975;86:781–2.

243. Rodriguez-Ruiz E, Martínez-Puga A, Carballo-Fazanes A, et al. Two new chest compression methods might challenge the standard in a simulated infant model. Eur J Pediatr 2019;178:1529–35.

244. Dorfsman ML, Menegazzi JJ, Wadas RJ, Auble TE. Two-thumb vs two-finger chest compression in an infant model of prolonged cardiopulmonary resuscitation. Acad Emerg Med 2000;7:1077–82.

245. Christman C, Hemway RJ, Wyckoff MH, Perlman JM. The two-thumb is superior to the two-finger method for administering chest compressions in a manikin model of neonatal resuscitation. Arch Dis Child Fetal Neonatal Ed 2011;96:F99–101.

246. Cheung PY, Huang H, Xu C, et al. Comparing the quality of cardiopulmonary resuscitation performed at the over-the-head position and lateral position of neonatal manikin. Front Pediatr 2020;7:559.

247. Phillips GW, Zideman DA. Relation of the infant heart to sternum: its significance in cardiopulmonary resuscitation. Lancet 1986;i:1024–5.

248. Finholt DA, Kettick RG, Wagner HR, et al. The heart is under the lower one third of the sternum. Am J Dis Child 1986;140:646–9.

249. Lee SH, Cho YC, Ryu S, et al. A comparison of the area of chest compression by the superimposed-thumb and the alongside-thumb techniques for infant cardiopulmonary resuscitation. Resuscitation 2011;82:1214–7.

250. Lim JS, Cho Y, Ryu S, et al. Comparison of overlapping (OP) and adjacent thumb positions (AP) for cardiac compressions using the encircling method in infants. Emerg Med J 2013;30:139–42.

251. Li ES, Cheung PY, O'Reilly M, Aziz K, Schmölzer GM. Rescuer fatigue during simulated neonatal cardiopulmonary resuscitation. J Perinatol 2015;35:142–5.

252. Solevåg AL, Cheung PY, O'Reilly M, Schmölzer GM. A review of approaches to optimise chest compressions in the resuscitation of asphyxiated newborns. Arch Dis Child Fetal Neonatal Ed 2016;101:F272–6.

253. Maher KO, Berg RA, Lindsey CW, et al. Depth of sternal compression and intra-arterial blood pressure during CPR in infants following cardiac surgery. Resuscitation 2009;80:662–4.

254. Meyer A, Nadkarni V, Pollock A, et al. Evaluation of the Neonatal Resuscitation Program's recommended chest compression depth using computerized tomography imaging. Resuscitation 2010;81:544–8.

255. Spevak MR, Kleinman PK, Belanger PL, et al. Cardiopulmonary resuscitation and rib fractures in infants; a postmortem radiologic pathologic study. JAMA 1994;272:617–8.

256. Dean JM, Koehler RC, Schleien CL, et al. Age-related effects of compression rate and duration in cardiopulmonary resuscitation. J Appl Physiol 1990;68:554–60.

257. Hemway RJ, Christman C, Perlman J. The 3:1 is superior to a 15:2 ratio in a newborn manikin model in terms of quality of chest compressions and number of ventilations. Arch Dis Child Fetal Neonatal Ed 2013;98:F42–5.

258. Solevåg AL, Madland JM, Gjærum E, Nakstad B. Minute ventilation at different compression to ventilation ratios, different ventilation rates, and continuous chest compressions with asynchronous ventilation in a newborn manikin. Scand J Trauma Resusc Emerg Med 2012;20:73.

259. Solevåg AL, Dannevig I, Wyckoff M, Saugstad OD, Nakstad B. Return of spontaneous circulation with a compression:ventilation ratio of 15:2 versus 3:1 in newborn pigs with cardiac arrest due to asphyxia. Arch Dis Child Fetal Neonatal Ed 2011;96:F417–21.

260. Whyte SD, Sinha AK, Wyllie JP. Neonatal resuscitation – a practical assessment. Resuscitation 1999;40:21–5.

261. Berg RA, Hilwig RW, Kern KB, Babar I, Ewy GA. Simulated mouth-to-mouth ventilation and chest compressions (bystander cardiopulmonary resuscitation) improves outcome in a swine model of prehospital pediatric asphyxia cardiac arrest. Crit Care Med 1999;27:1893–9.

262. Idris AH, Becker LB, Fuerst RS, et al. Effect of ventilation on resuscitation in an animal model of cardiac arrest. Circulation 1994;90:3063–9.

263. Linner R, Werner O, Perez-de-Sa V, Cunha-Goncalves D. Circulatory recovery is as fast with air ventilation as with 100% oxygen after asphyxia-induced cardiac arrest in piglets. Pediatr Res 2009;66:391–4.

264. Solevåg AL, Dannevig I, Nakstad B, Saugstad OD. Resuscitation of severely asphyctic newborn pigs with cardiac arrest by using 21% or 100% oxygen. Neonatology 2010;98:64–72.

265. Temesvári P, Karg E, Bódi I, et al. Impaired early neurologic outcome in newborn piglets reoxygenated with 100% oxygen compared with room air after pneumothorax-induced asphyxia. Pediatr Res 2001;49:812–9.

266. Schmölzer GM, O'Reilly M, Labossiere J, et al. 3:1 compression to ventilation ratio versus continuous chest compression with asynchronous ventilation in a porcine model of neonatal resuscitation. Resuscitation 2014;85:270–5.

267. Sims DG, Heal CA, Bartle SM. The use of adrenaline and atropine in neonatal resuscitation. Arch Dis Child Fetal Neonatal Ed 1994;70: F3–10.

268. O'Donnell AI, Gray PH, Rogers YM. Mortality and neurodevelopmental outcome for infants receiving adrenaline in neonatal resuscitation. J Paediatr Child Health 1988;34:551–6.

269. Ellemunter H, Simma B, Trawoger R, Maurer H. Intraosseous lines in preterm and full term neonates. Arch Dis Child Fetal Neonatal Ed 1999;80:F74–5.

270. Scrivens A, Reynolds PR, Emery FE, et al. Use of intraosseous needles in neonates: a systematic review. Neonatology 2019;116:305–14.

271. Costa S, De Carolis MP, Savarese I, et al. An unusual complication of umbilical catheterisation. Eur J Pediatr 2008;167:1467–9.

272. Lindemann R. Resuscitation of the newborn with endotracheal administration of epinephrine. Acta Paed Scand 1984;73:210–2.

273. Isayama T, Mildenhall L, Schmölzer GM, et al; International Liaison Committee On Resuscitation Newborn Life Support Task Force. The route, dose, and interval of epinephrine for neonatal resuscitation: a systematic review. Pediatrics 2020;146:e20200586.

274. Diamond LK, Allen FH Jr, Thomas WO Jr. Erythroblastosis fetalis. VII. Treatment with exchange transfusion. N Engl J Med 1951;244:39–49.

275. Hall RT, Rhodes PG. Total parenteral alimentation via indwelling umbilical catheters in the newborn period. Arch Dis Child 1976;51:929–34.

276. Linde LM, Higashino SM, Berman G, et al. Umbilical vessel cardiac catheterization and angiocardiography. Circulation 1966;34:984–8.

277. Prinz SC, Cunningham MD. Umbilical vessel catheterization. J Fam Pract 1980;10:885–90.

278. Pinto M, Solevåg AL, O'Reilly M, et al. Evidence on adrenaline use in resuscitation and its relevance to newborn infants: a non-systematic review. Neonatology 2017;111:37–44.

279. Michael JR, Guerci AD, Koehler RC, et al. Mechanisms by which epinephrine augments cerebral and myocardial perfusion during cardiopulmonary resuscitation in dogs. Circulation 1984;69:822–35.

280. Paradis NA, Martin GB, Rivers EP, et al. Coronary perfusion pressure and the return of spontaneous circulation in human cardiopulmonary resuscitation. JAMA 1990;263:1106–13.

281. Redding JS, Pearson JW. Evaluation of drugs for cardiac resuscitation. Anesthesiology 1963;24:203–7.

282. Brown CG, Werman HA, Davis EA, et al. The effects of graded doses of epinephrine on regional myocardial flow during cardiopulmonary resuscitation in swine. Circulation 1987;75:491–7.

283. Lindner KH, Ahnefeld FW, Bowdler IM. Comparison of different doses of epinephrine on myocardial perfusion and resuscitation success during cardiopulmonary resuscitation in a pig model. Am J Emerg Med 1991;9:27–31.

284. Perondi MB, Reis AG, Paiva EF, et al. A comparison of high-dose and standard-dose epinephrine in children with cardiac arrest. N Engl J Med 2004;350:1722–30.

285. Berg RA, Otto CW, Kern KB, et al. A randomized, blinded trial of high dose epinephrine versus standard-dose epinephrine in a swine model of pediatric asphyxial cardiac arrest. Crit Care Med 1996;24:1695–700.

286. Pasternak JF, Groothius DR, Fisher DP. Regional cerebral blood flow in the beagle puppy model of neonatal intraventricular hemorrhage: studies in systemic hypertension. Neurology 1983;33:559–66.

287. Modest VE, Butterworth JF 4th. Effect of pH and lidocaine on betaadrenergic receptor binding: interaction during resuscitation. Chest 1995;108:1373–9.

288. Redding JS, Asuncion JS, Pearson JW. Effective routes of drug administration during cardiac arrest. Anesth Analg (Clev) 1967;46:253–8.

289. Halling C, Sparks JE, Christie L, Wyckoff MH. Efficacy of intravenous and endotracheal epinephrine during neonatal cardiopulmonary resuscitation in the delivery room. J Pediatr 2017;185:232–6.

290. Vali P, Chandrasekharan P, Rawat M, et al. Evaluation of timing and route of epinephrine in a neonatal model of asphyxial arrest. J Am Heart Assoc 2017;6:e004402.

291. Basu P, Som S, Choudhuri N, et al. Contribution of the blood glucose level in perinatal asphyxia. Eur J Pediatr 2009;168:833–8.

292. Azzopardi D, Strohm B, Linsell L, et al; UK TOBY Cooling Register. Implementation and conduct of therapeutic hypothermia for perinatal asphyxial encephalopathy in the UK – analysis of national data. PLoS One 2012;7:e38504.

293. Basu SK, Kaiser JR, Guffey D, et al; CoolCap Study Group. Hypoglycaemia and hyperglycaemia are associated with unfavourable outcome in infants with hypoxic ischaemic encephalopathy: a post hoc analysis of the CoolCap Study. Arch Dis Child Fetal Neonatal Ed 2016;101:F149–55.

294. Basu SK, Ottolini K, Govindan V, et al. Early glycemic profile is associated with brain injury patterns on magnetic resonance imaging in hypoxic ischemic encephalopathy. J Pediatr 2018;203:137–43.

295. Aslam A, Vincer M, Allen A, Imanullah S, O'Connell CM. Long-term outcomes of saline boluses in very preterm infants. J Neonatal Perinatal Med 2018;11:317–21.

296. Skellet S, Mayer A, Durward A, et al. Chasing the base deficit: hyperchloraemic acidosis following 0.9% saline fluid resuscitation. Arch Dis Child 2000;83:514–6.

297. Aschner JL, Poland RL. Sodium bicarbonate: basically useless therapy. Pediatrics 2008;122:831–5.

298. Smith GC. Life-table analysis of the risk of perinatal death at term and post term in singleton pregnancies. Am J Obstet Gynecol 2001;184:489–96.

299. Stanley FJ, Alberman ED. Infants of very low birthweight. 1. Factors affecting survival. Dev Med Child Neurol 1978;20:300–12.

300. Merritt TA, Farrell PM. Diminished pulmonary lecithin synthesis in acidosis: Experimental findings as related to the respiratory distress syndrome. Pediatrics 1976;57:32–40.

301. Bensouda B, Mandel R, Mejri A, et al. Temperature probe placement during preterm infant resuscitation: a randomised trial. Neonatology 2018;113:27–32.

302. Reilly MC, Vohra S, Rac VE, et al; Vermont Oxford Network Heat Loss Prevention (HeLP) Trial Study Group. Randomized trial of occlusive wrap for heat loss prevention in preterm infants. J Pediatr 2015;166:262–8.e2.

303. Meyer MP, Owen LS, Te Pas AB. Use of heated humidified gases for early stabilization of preterm infants: a meta-analysis. Front Pediatr 2018;6:319.

304. Li S, Guo P, Zou Q, et al. Efficacy and safety of plastic wrap for prevention of hypothermia after birth and during NICU in preterm infants: a systematic review and meta-analysis. PLoS One 2016;11:e0156960.

305. Belsches TC, Tilly AE, Miller TR, et al. Randomized trial of plastic bags to prevent term neonatal hypothermia in a resource-poor setting. Pediatrics 2013;132:e656–61.

306. Leadford AE, Warren JB, Manasyan A, et al. Plastic bags for prevention of hypothermia in preterm and low birth weight infants. Pediatrics 2013;132:e128–34.

307. Björklund LJ, Ingimarsson J, Curstedt T, et al. Manual ventilation with a few large breaths at birth compromises the therapeutic effect of subsequent surfactant replacement in immature lambs. Pediatr Res 1997;42:348–55.

308. Schmölzer GM, Kamlin OC, O'Donnell CP, et al. Assessment of tidal volume and gas leak during mask ventilation of preterm infants in the delivery room. Arch Dis Child Fetal Neonatal Ed 2010;95:F393–7.

309. O'Donnell CP, Kamlin CO, Davis PG, Morley CJ. Crying and breathing by extremely preterm infants immediately after birth. J Pediatr 2010;156:846–7.

310. Schmölzer GM, Kumar M, Pichler G, et al. Non-invasive versus invasive respiratory support in preterm infants at birth: systematic review and meta-analysis. Brit Med J 2013;347:f5980.

311. O'Currain E, O'Shea JE, McGrory L, et al. Smaller facemasks for positive pressure ventilation in preterm infants: A randomised trial. Resuscitation 2019;134:91–8.

312. Kuypers KL, Lamberska T, Martherus T, et al. The effect of a face mask for respiratory support on breathing in preterm infants at birth. Resuscitation 2019;144:178–84.

313. Kuypers K, Martherus T, Lamberska T, et al. Reflexes that impact spontaneous breathing of preterm infants at birth: a narrative review. Arch Dis Child Fetal Neonatal Ed 2020;105:F675–9.

314. Crawshaw JR, Kitchen MJ, Binder-Heschl C, et al. Laryngeal closure impedes non-invasive ventilation at birth. Arch Dis Child Fetal Neonatal Ed 2018;103:F112–9.

315. Morley CJ, Davis PG, Doyle L, et al. Nasal CPAP or intubation for very preterm infants. New Engl J Med 2008;358:700–8.

316. Ingimarsson J, Björklund LJ, Curstedt T. Incomplete protection by prophylactic surfactant against the adverse effects of large lung inflation in immature lambs at birth. Intensive Care Med 2004;30:1446–53.

317. Andresen JH, Saugstad OD. Oxygen metabolism and oxygenation of the newborn. Semin Fetal Neonatal Med 2020;25:101078.

318. Kapadia V, Oei JL. Optimizing oxygen therapy for preterm infants at birth: Are we there yet? Semin Fetal Neonatal Med 2020;25:101081.

319. Welsford M, Nishiyama C, Shortt C, et al; on behalf of the International Liaison Committee on Resuscitation Neonatal Life Support Task Force. Initial oxygen use for preterm newborn resuscitation: a systematic review with meta-analysis. Pediatrics 2019;143:e20181828.

320. Schmölzer GM, Kamlin COF, Dawson JA, et al. Respiratory monitoring of neonatal resuscitation. Arch Dis Child Fetal Neonatal Ed 2010;95:F295–303.

321. Mian QN, Pichler G, Binder C, et al. Tidal volumes in spontaneously breathing preterm infants supported with continuous positive airway pressure. J Pediatr 2014;165:702–6.e1.

322. Poulton DA, Schmölzer GM, Morley CJ, Davis PG. Assessment of chest rise during mask ventilation of preterm infants in the delivery room. Resuscitation 2011;82:175–9.

323. Verder H, Albertsen P, Ebbesen F. et al. Nasal continuous positive airway pressure and early surfactant therapy for respiratory distress syndrome in newborns of less than 30 weeks gestation. Pediatrics 1999;103:e24.

324. Birch S, Rhodes H, Wylie P. Laryngeal damage from intubation (case report). Br Med J 1999;318:614.

325. Rojas-Reyes MX, Morley CJ, Soll R. Prophylactic versus selective use of surfactant in preventing morbidity and mortality in preterm infants. Cochrane Database Syst Rev 2012;3:CD000510.

326. Panza R, Laforgia N, Bellos I, Pandita A. Systematic review found that using thin catheters to deliver surfactant to preterm neonates was associated with reduced bronchopulmonary dysplasia and mechanical ventilation. Acta Paediatr 2020;109:2219–25.

327. Calevo MG, Veronese N, Cavallin F, et al. Supraglottic airway devices for surfactant treatment: systematic review and meta-analysis. J Perinatol 2019;39:173–83.

328. Oei JL, Kapadia V. Oxygen for respiratory support of moderate and late preterm and term infants at birth: Is air best? Semin Fetal Neonatal Med 2020;25:101074.

329. Hadar A, Rabinovich A, Sheiner E, et al. Obstetric characteristics and neonatal outcome of unplanned out-of-hospital term deliveries: a prospective, case-control study. J Reprod Med 2005;50:832–6.

330. Brocklehurst P, Hardy P, Hollowell J, et al; Birthplace in England Collaborative Group. Perinatal and maternal outcomes by planned place of birth for healthy women with low risk pregnancies: the Birthplace in England national prospective cohort study. Brit Med J 2011;343:d7400.

331. de Groene L, De Jaegere AP, Nijland OJ, van Kaam AH. Validation of the disposable T-piece resuscitator (Neo-Tee): a bench study. Arch Dis Child Fetal Neonatal Ed 2019;104:F594–7.

332. Trevisanuto D, Verghese C, Doglioni N, et al. Laryngeal mask airway for the interhospital transport of neonates. Pediatrics 2005;115:e109–11.

333. McLelland GE, Morgans AE, McKenna LG. Involvement of emergency medical services at unplanned births before arrival to hospital: a structured review. Emerg Med J 2014;31:345–50.

334. Adamsons K Jr, Behrman R, Dawes GS, et al. Resuscitation by positive pressure ventilation and Tris-hydroxymethyl-aminomethane in rhesus monkeys asphyxiated at birth. J Pediatr 1964;65:807–18.

335. Okumura A, Hayakawa F, Kato T, et al. Hypocarbia in preterm infants with periventricular leukomalacia: the relation between hypocarbia and mechanical ventilation. Pediatrics 2001;107:469–75.

336. Sweet DG, Carnielli V, Greisen G, et al. European Consensus Guidelines on the Management of Respiratory Distress Syndrome - 2019 Update. Neonatology 2019;115:432–50.

337. Akinloye O, O'Connell C, Allen AC, El-Naggar W. Post-resuscitation care for neonates receiving positive pressure ventilation at birth. Pediatrics 2014;134:e1057–62.

338. Holme H, Bhatt R, Koumettou M, Griffin MA, Winckworth LC. Retrospective evaluation of a new neonatal trigger score. Pediatrics 2013;131:e837–42.

339. Roland D, Madar J, Connolly G. The Newborn Early Warning (NEW) system: development of an at-risk infant intervention system. Infant 2010;6:116–20.

340. Natarajan G, Pappas A, Shankaran S. Outcomes in childhood following therapeutic hypothermia for neonatal hypoxic-ischemic encephalopathy (HIE). Semin Perinatol 2016;40:549–55.

341. Lamblin MD, Walls Esquivel E, André M. The electroencephalogram of the full-term newborn: review of normal features and hypoxic-ischemic encephalopathy patterns. Neurophysiol Clin 2013;43:267–87.

342. Hutton EK, Thorpe J. Consequences of meconium stained amniotic fluid: what does the evidence tell us? Early Hum Dev 2014;90:333–9.

343. Cabal LA, Devaskar U, Siassi B, et al. Cardiogenic shock associated with perinatal asphyxia in preterm infants. J Pediatr 1980;96:705–10.

344. Ahearne CE, Boylan GB, Murray DM. Short and long term prognosis in perinatal asphyxia: An update. World J Clin Pediatr 2016;5:67–74.

345. Eunson P. The long-term health, social, and financial burden of hypoxic-ischaemic encephalopathy. Dev Med Child Neurol 2015;57 (Suppl 3):48–50.

346. Westgate J, Garibaldi JM, Greene KR. Umbilical cord blood gas analysis at delivery: a time for quality data. Br J Obstet Gynaecol 1994;101:1054–63.

347. Goldenberg RL, Huddleston JF, Nelson KG. Apgar scores and umbilical arterial pH in preterm infants. Am J Obstet Gynecol 1984;149:651–4.

348. Johnson JWC, Richards DS, Wagaman RA. The case for routine umbilical blood acid-base studies at delivery. Am J Obstet Gynecol 1990;162:621–5.

349. Tong S, Egan V, Griffin J, Wallace EM. Cord blood sampling at delivery: do we need to always collect from both vessels? BJOG 2002;109:1175-7.

350. Armstrong L, Stenson B. The effect of delayed sampling on umbilical cord arterial and venous lactate and blood gases in clamped and unclamped vessels. Arch Dis Child Fetal Neonatal Ed 2006;91:F342–5.

351. Wong L, MacLennan AH. Gathering the evidence: cord gases and placental histology for births with low Apgar scores. Aust N Z J Obstet Gynaecol 2011;51:17–21.

352. Pelikan DM, Scherjon SA, Kanhai HH. The incidence of large fetomaternal hemorrhage and the Kleihauer-Betke test. Obstet Gynecol 2005;106:642–3.

353. National Institute for Health and Care Excellence. Neonatal infection (early onset): antibiotics for prevention and treatment. NICE Clinical guideline [CG149], 2012.

354. Kurinczuk JJ, White-Koning M, Badawi N. Epidemiology of neonatal encephalopathy and hypoxic-ischaemic encephalopathy. Early Hum Dev 2010;86:329–38.

355. Department of Health. An organisation with a memory. Report of an expert group on learning from adverse events in the NHS, chaired by the Chief Medical Officer. London: The Stationery Office; 2000.

356. Azzopardi D, Strohm B, Edwards AD, et al. Moderate hypothermia to treat perinatal asphyxial encephalopathy. N Engl J Med 2009;361:1349–58.

357. National Institute for Health and Care Excellence (NICE). Therapeutic hypothermia with intracorporeal temperature monitoring for hypoxic perinatal brain injury: guidance. NICE interventional procedure guidance [IPG347]. London, 2010.

358. BAPM. Therapeutic Hypothermia for Neonatal Encephalopathy; A Framework for Practice. British Association of Perinatal Medicine, London, 2020.

359. Jacobs SE, Berg M, Hunt R, et al. Cooling for newborns with hypoxic ischaemic encephalopathy. Cochrane Database Syst Rev 2013;1:CD003311.

360. Kasdorf E, Perlman JM. Hyperthermia, inflammation, and perinatal brain injury. Pediatr Neurol 2013;49:8–14.

361. Kendall GS, Kapetanakis A, Ratnavel N, et al. Passive cooling for initiation of therapeutic hypothermia in neonatal encephalopathy. Arch Dis Child Fetal Neonatal Ed 2010;95:F408–12.

362. Leahy FAN, Cates D, MacCallum M, Rigatto H. Effect of CO2 and 100% O2 on cerebral blood flow in preterm infants. J Appl Physiol 1980;48:468–72.

363. Klinger G, Beyene J, Shah P, Perlman M. Do hyperoxaemia and hypercapnia add to the risk of brain injury after intrapartum asphyxia? Arch Dis Child Fetal Neonatal Ed 2005;90:49–52.

364. Ainsworth SB. Neonatal Formulary: Drug Use in Pregnancy and the First Year of Life. 8th edition. Oxford University Press, Oxford, 2020. pp. 46–49.

365. Madar J. Clinical risk management in newborn and neonatal resuscitation. Semin Fetal Neonatal Med 2005;10:45–61.

366. Schilleman K, Witlox RS, van Vonderen JJ, et al. Auditing documentation on delivery room management using video and physiological recordings. Arch Dis Child Fetal Neonatal Ed 2014;99:F485–90.

367. Berglund S, Norman M. Neonatal resuscitation assessment: documentation and early paging must be improved! Arch Dis Child Fetal Neonatal Ed 2012;97:F204–8.

368. Cavallin F , Pavan G , Cavicchiolo ME , et al. Multicentre study found that documentation on resuscitating asphyxiated neonates was often unsatisfactory. Acta Paediatr 2019;108:562–3.

369. Fishman CE, Weinberg DD, Murray A, Foglia EE. Accuracy of real-time delivery room resuscitation documentation. Arch Dis Child Fetal Neonatal Ed 2020;105:222–4.

370. NMC. The Code: Professional standards of practice and behaviour for nurses, midwives and nursing associates. Nursing & Midwifery Council, London 2015 (updated 2018).

371. GMC. Good Medical Practice; Record your work clearly, accurately and legibly. Domain 1; points 19–21. General Medical Council, London, 2013.

372. Mead J. Paediatricians negligent in emergency: Antoniades v East Sussex Hospitals NHS Trust (High Court, 16/03/07 - Mackay J). Clin Risk 2008;14:82–3.

373. Ewer AK, Middleton LJ, Furmston AT, et al; PulseOx Study Group. Pulse oximetry screening for congenital heart defects in newborn infants (PulseOx): a test accuracy study. Lancet 2011;378:785–94.

374. Morland TA, Brice JEM, Walker CHM, Parija AC. Naloxone pharmacokinetics in the newborn. Br J Clin Pharmacol 1979;9:609–12.

375. Shah P, Anvekar A, McMichael J, Rao S. Outcomes of infants with Apgar score of zero at 10 min: the West Australian experience. Arch Dis Child Fetal Neonatal Ed 2015;100:F492–4.

376. Zhong YJ, Claveau M, Yoon EW, et al; Canadian Neonatal Network (CNN) Investigators. Neonates with a 10-min Apgar score of zero: Outcomes by gestational age. Resuscitation 2019;143:77–84.

377. Zhang SQ, Friedman H, Strand ML. Length of resuscitation for severely depressed newborns. Am J Perinatol 2020;37:933–8.

378. Torke AM, Bledsoe P, Wocial LD, et al. CEASE: a guide for clinicians on how to stop resuscitation efforts. Ann Am Thorac Soc 2015;12:440–5.

379. Foglia EE, Weiner G, de Almeida MFB, et al; International Liaison Committee on Resuscitation Neonatal Life Support Task Force. Duration of resuscitation at birth, mortality, and neurodevelopment: a systematic review. Pediatrics 2020;146:e20201449.

380. Pyle AK, Fleischman AR, Hardart G, Mercurio MR. Management options and parental voice in the treatment of trisomy 13 and 18. J Perinatol 2018;38:1135–43.

381. Winn P, Acharya K, Peterson E, Leuthner S. Prenatal counseling and parental decision-making following a fetal diagnosis of trisomy 13 or 18. J Perinatol 2018;38:788–96.

382. Wilkinson DJ, Thiele P, Watkins A, De Crespigny L. Fatally flawed? A review and ethical analysis of lethal congenital malformations. BJOG 2012;119:1302–8.

383. Macfarlane PI, Wood S, Bennett J. Non-viable delivery at 20-23 weeks gestation: observations and signs of life after birth. Arch Dis Child Fetal Neonatal Ed 2003;88:F199–202.

384. Garten L, Bührer C. Pain and distress management in palliative neonatal care. Semin Fetal Neonatal Med 2019;24:101008.

385. Royal College of Paediatrics and Child Health. Withholding or withdrawing life sustaining treatment in children—a framework for practice. 2nd edn. London: RCPCH, 2004.

386. Thomas EJ, Williams AL, Reichman EF, et al. Team training in the neonatal resuscitation program for interns: teamwork and quality of resuscitations. Pediatrics 2010;125:539–46.

387. Williams AL, Lasky RE, Dannemiller JL, et al. Teamwork behaviours and errors during neonatal resuscitation. Qual Saf Health Care 2010;19:60–4.

388. Katakam LI, Trickey AW, Thomas EJ. Speaking up and sharing information improves trainee neonatal resuscitations. J Patient Saf 2012;8:202–9.

389. Catchpole K. Cited in department of health human factors reference group interim report, 1 March 2012, National Quality Board. March 2012. (available at www.england.nhs.uk/wp-content/uploads/2013/11/DH-rep.pdf - accessed 30 January 2021)

390. Clarkson J, Dean J, Ward J, Komashie A, Bashford T. A systems approach to healthcare: from thinking to practice. Future Healthc J 2018;5:151–5.

391. Maskery S. Neonatal resuscitation. Clin Risk 2008;14:46–8.

392. Plaat F. The team needs a leader. Clin Risk 2008;14:43–5.

393. Thomas EJ, Sexton JB, Lasky RE, et al. Teamwork and quality during neonatal care in the delivery room. J Perinatol 2006;26:163–9.

394. Salih ZNI, Draucker CB. Facilitators of and barriers to successful teamwork during resuscitations in a neonatal intensive care unit. J Perinatol 2019;39:974–82.

395. Greig PR, Higham H, Nobre AC. Failure to perceive clinical events: An under-recognised source of error. Resuscitation 2014;85:952–6.

396. Goleman D. Leadership that gets results. Harvard Business Review 2000;March–April:79–90.

397. Norris EM, Lockey AS. Human factors in resuscitation teaching. Resuscitation 2012;83:423–7.

398. Yamada NK, Halamek LP. On the need for precise, concise communication during resuscitation: a proposed solution. J Pediatr 2015;166:184–7.

399. Riskin A, Erez A, Foulk TA, et al. The impact of rudeness on medical team performance: a randomized trial. Pediatrics 2015;136:487–95.

400. Thomas EJ, Taggart B, Crandell S, et al. Teaching teamwork during the Neonatal Resuscitation Program: a randomized trial. J Perinatol 2007;27:409–14.

401. Kohn LT, Corrigan JM, Donaldson MS eds. To Err is Human. Building a Safer Health System. Washington, DC: National Academy Press, 1999. (full text available on-line at https://www.nap.edu/catalog/9728/to-err-is-human-building-a-safer-health-system)

402. Halamek LP, Cady RAH, Sterling MR. Using briefing, simulation and debriefing to improve human and system performance. Semin Perinatol 2019;43:151178.

403. Mosley CM, Shaw BN. A longitudinal cohort study to investigate the retention of knowledge and skills following attendance on the Newborn Life support course. Arch Dis Child 2013;98:582–6.

404. Couper K, Perkins GD. Debriefing after resuscitation. Curr Opin Crit Care 2013;19:188–94.

405. Allbutt C. Diseases of the arteries including angina pectoris, vol 1. London: Macmillan, 1915, p 154.

406. Editorial. Anoxia in the newborn. Lancet 1951;ii:821–2.

407. Carson BS, Losey RW, Bowes WA Jr, Simmons MA. Combined obstetric and pediatric approach to prevent meconium aspiration syndrome. Am J Obstet Gynecol 1976;126:712–5.

408. Daga SR, Dave K, Mehta V, Pai V. Tracheal suction in meconium stained infants: a randomized controlled study. J Trop Pediatr 1994;40:198–200.

409. Linder N, Aranda JV, Tsur M, et al. Need for endotracheal intubation and suction in meconium-stained neonates. J Pediatr 1988;112:613–5.

410. Liu WF, Harrington T. The need for delivery room intubation of thin meconium in the low-risk newborn: a clinical trial. Am J Perinatol 1998;15:675–82.

411. Kumar A, Kumar P, Basu S. Endotracheal suctioning for prevention of meconium aspiration syndrome: a randomized controlled trial. Eur J Pediatr 2019;178:1825–32.

412. Finer NN, Carlo WA, Walsh MC, et al. Early CPAP versus surfactant in extremely preterm infants. N Engl J Med 2010;362:1970–9.

413. Dunn MS, Kaempf J, de Klerk A, et al. Randomized trial comparing 3 approaches to the initial respiratory management of preterm neonates. Pediatrics 2011;128:e1069–76.

414. Subramaniam P, Ho JJ, Davis PG. Prophylactic nasal continuous positive airway pressure for preventing morbidity and mortality in very preterm infants. Cochrane Database Syst Rev 2016;6:CD001243.

415. Konstantelos D, Ifflaender S, Dinger J, Burkhardt W, Rüdiger M. Analyzing support of postnatal transition in term infants after c-section. BMC Pregnancy Childbirth 2014;14:225.

416. Hein HA. The use of sodium bicarbonate in neonatal resuscitation: help or harm. Pediatrics 1993;91:496–7.

417. Kapadia VS, Wyckoff MH. Drugs during delivery room resuscitation--what, when and why? Semin Fetal Neonatal Med 2013;18:357-61.

418. Sáenz P, Brugada M, de Jongh B, et al. A survey of intravenous sodium bicarbonate in neonatal asphyxia among European neonatologists: gaps between scientific evidence and clinical practice. Neonatology 2011;99:170–6.

419. Lokesh L, Kumar P, Murki S, et al. A randomized controlled trial of sodium bicarbonate in neonatal resuscitation: effect on immediate outcome. Resuscitation 2004;60:219–23.

420. Murki S, Kumar P, Lingappa L, et al. Effect of a single dose of sodium bicarbonate given during neonatal resuscitation at birth on the acid—base status on first day of life. J Perinatol 2004;24,696–9.

421. Preziosi MP, Roig JC, Hargrove N, et al. Metabolic acidemia with hypoxia attenuates the haemodynamic responses to epinephrine during resuscitation in lambs. Crit Care Med 1993;21:1901–7.

422. Raymondos K, Panning B, Leuwer M, et al. Absorption and hemodynamic effects of airway administration of adrenaline in patients with severe cardiac disease. Ann Intern Med 2000;132:800–3.

423. Kleinman ME, Oh W, Stonstreet BS. Comparison of intravenous and endotracheal epinephrine during cardiopulmonary resuscitation in newborn piglets. Crit Care Med 1999;27:2748–85.

424. Crespo SG, Schoffstall JM, Fuhs LR, Spivey WH. Comparison of two doses of endotracheal epinephrine in a cardiac arrest model. Ann Emerg Med 1991;20:230–4.

425. Jasani MS, Nadkarni VM, Finkelstein MS, et al. Effects of different techniques of endotracheal epinephrine administration in pediatric porcine hypoxic-hypercarbic cardiopulmonary arrest. Crit Care Med 1994;22:1174–80.

426. Nair J, Vali P, Gugino SF, et al. Bioavailability of endotracheal epinephrine in an ovine model of neonatal resuscitation. Early Hum Dev 2019;130:27–32.

427. Gibbs J, Newson T, Williams J, Davidson DC. Naloxone hazard in infant of opioid abuser. Lancet 1989;ii:159–60.

428. Deshpande G, Gill A. Cardiac arrest following naloxone in an extremely preterm neonate. Eur J Pediatr 2009;168:115–7.

429. Martinez A, Padbury J, Shames L, Evans C, Humme J. Naloxone potentiates epinephrine release during hypoxia in fetal sheep: dose response and cardiovascular effects. Pediatr Res 1988;23:343–7.

430. Padbury JF, Agata Y, Polk DH, Wang DL, Callegari CC. Neonatal adaptation: naloxone increases the catecholamine surge at birth. Pediatr Res 1987;21:590–3.

431. McGuire W, Fowlie PW. Naloxone for narcotic exposed newborn infants: systematic review. Arch Dis Child Fetal Neonatal Ed 2003;88:F308–11.

432. Moe-Byrne T, Brown JVE, McGuire W. Naloxone for opioid-exposed newborn infants. Cochrane Database Syst Rev 2018;10:CD003483.

433. Granfeldt A, Avis SR, Lind PC, et al. Intravenous vs. intraosseous administration of drugs during cardiac arrest: A systematic review. Resuscitation 2020;149:150–7.

434. Gupta N, Corbett H, Ismail R, et al. Allantoic cyst - an unusual umbilical cord swelling. J Surg Case Rep 2011;2011:5.

435. Mattei P. Urachal remnant perforation during umbilical vein catheterization in a newborn. J Pediatr Surg 2007;42:722–4.

436. Robinson JN, Abuhamad AZ. Abdominal wall and umbilical cord anomalies. Clin Perinatol 2000;27:947–78.

437. Rajani AK, Chitkara R, Oehlert J, et al. Comparison of umbilical venous and intraosseous access during simulated neonatal resuscitation. Pediatrics 2011;128:e954–8.

438. Karlberg P, Koch G. Respiratory studies in newborn infants. III. Development of mechanics of breathing during the first week of life. A longitudinal study. Acta Paediatr Suppl 1962;135:121–9.

439. Vyas H, Field D, Milner AD, Hopkin IE. Determinants of the first inspiratory volume and functional residual capacity at birth. Pediatr Pulmonol 1986;2:189–93.

440. te Pas AB, Wong C, Kamlin CO, Dawson JA, Morley CJ, Davis PG. Breathing patterns in preterm and term infants immediately after birth. Pediatr Res 2009;65:352–6.

441. Bruschettini M, O'Donnell CP, Davis PG, Morley CJ, Moja L, Calevo MG. Sustained versus standard inflations during neonatal resuscitation to prevent mortality and improve respiratory outcomes. Cochrane Database Syst Rev 2020;3:CD004953.

442. Lindner W, Högel J, Pohlandt F. Sustained pressure-controlled inflation or intermittent mandatory ventilation in preterm infants in the delivery room? A randomized, controlled trial on initial respiratory support via nasopharyngeal tube. Acta Paediatr 2005;94:303–9.

443. Lista G, Boni L, Scopesi F, et al; SLI trial investigators. Sustained lung inflation at birth for preterm infants: a randomized clinical trial. Pediatrics 2015;135:e457–64.

444. Schwaberger B, Pichler G, Avian A, Binder-Heschl C, Baik N, Urlesberger B. Do sustained lung inflations during neonatal resuscitation affect cerebral blood volume in preterm infants? A randomized controlled pilot study. PLoS One 2015;10:e0138964.

445. Mercadante D, Colnaghi M, Polimeni V, et al. Sustained lung inflation in late preterm infants: a randomized controlled trial. J Perinatol 2016;36:443–7.

446. Abd El-Fattah N, Nasef N, Al-Harrass MF, Khashaba M. Sustained lung inflation at birth for preterm infants at risk of respiratory distress syndrome: The proper pressure and duration. J Neonatal Perinatal Med 2017;10:409-417.

447. El-Chimi MS, Awad HA, El-Gammasy TM, El-Farghali OG, Sallam MT, Shinkar DM. Sustained versus intermittent lung inflation for resuscitation of preterm infants: a randomized controlled trial. J Matern Fetal Neonatal Med 2017;30:1273–8.

448. Jiravisitkul P, Rattanasiri S, Nuntnarumit P. Randomised controlled trial of sustained lung inflation for resuscitation of preterm infants in the delivery room. Resuscitation 2017;111:68–73.

449. Ngan AY, Cheung PY, Hudson-Mason A, et al. Using exhaled CO2 to guide initial respiratory support at birth: a randomised controlled trial. Arch Dis Child Fetal Neonatal Ed 2017;102:F525–31.

450. Schmölzer GM, O Reilly M, Fray C, van Os S, Cheung PY. Chest compression during sustained inflation versus 3:1 chest compression:ventilation ratio during neonatal cardiopulmonary resuscitation: a randomised feasibility trial. Arch Dis Child Fetal Neonatal Ed 2018;103:F455–60.

451. Yeomans ER, Hauth JC, Gilstrap LC 3rd, et al. Umbilical cord pH, PCO2, and bicarbonate following uncomplicated term vaginal deliveries. Am J Obstet Gynecol 1985;151:798–800.

452. Gilstrap LC 3rd, Leveno KJ, Burris J, et al. Diagnosis of birth asphyxia on the basis of fetal pH, Apgar score, and newborn cerebral dysfunction. Am J Obstet Gynecol 1989;161:825–30.

453. Fee SC, Malee K, Deddish R, et al. Severe acidosis and subsequent neurologic status. Am J Obstet Gynecol 1990;162:802–6.

454. Wiberg N, Källén K, Herbst A, Olofsson P. Relation between umbilical cord blood pH, base deficit, lactate, 5-minute Apgar score and development of hypoxic ischemic encephalopathy. Acta Obstet Gynecol Scand 2010;89:1263-9.

455. James LS, Weisbrot IM, Prince CE, et al. The acid base status of human infants in relation to birth asphyxia and the onset of respiration. J Pediatr 1958;52:379–94.

456. Martin GC, Green RS, Holzman IR. Acidosis in newborns with nuchal cords and normal Apgar scores. J Perinatol 2005;25:162–5.

457. Johnson JW, Richards DS. The etiology of fetal acidosis as determined by umbilical cord acid-base studies. Am J Obstet Gynecol 1997;177:274–80.

458. Pomerance J. Umbilical cord blood gases casebook. Interpreting umbilical cord blood gases, VII. J Perinatol 2000;20:338–9.

459. Giovannini N, Crippa BL, Denaro E, et al. The effect of delayed umbilical cord clamping on cord blood gas analysis in vaginal and caesarean-delivered term newborns without fetal distress: a prospective observational study. BJOG 2020;127:405–13.

460. Apgar V. A proposal for a new method of evaluation of the newborn infant. Anesth Analg (Clev) 1953;32:260–7.

461. Apgar V, James LS. Further observations on the Newborn Scoring System. Am J Dis Child 1962;104:419–28.

462. Lie KK, Groholt EK, Eskild A. Association of cerebral palsy with Apgar score in low and normal birthweight infants – a population based cohort study. Br Med J 2010;341:c4990.

463. Nelson KB, Ellenberg JH. Apgar scores as predictors of chronic neurological disability. Pediatrics 1981;68:36–44.

464. Sykes G, Molloy P, Johnson P, et al. Do Apgar scores indicate asphyxia? Lancet 1982;i:494–6.

465. Power BD, McGinley J, Sweetman D, Murphy JFA. The modified Sarnat score in the assessment of neonatal encephalopathy: A quality improvement initiative. Ir Med J 2019;112:976.

466. Robertson CMT, Finer NN, Grace MGA. School performance in survivors of neonatal encephalopathy associated with birth asphyxia at term. J Pediatr 1989;114:753–60.

467. Cui J, Li F, Shi ZL. Origin and evolution of pathogenic coronaviruses. Nat Rev Microbiol 2019;17:181–92.

468. Chandrasekharan P, Vento M, Trevisanuto D, et al. Neonatal resuscitation and postresuscitation care of infants born to mothers with suspected or confirmed SARS-CoV-2 infection. Am J Perinatol 2020;37:813–24.

469. Shiu EYC, Leung NHL, Cowling BJ. Controversy around airborne versus droplet transmission of respiratory viruses: implication for infection prevention. Curr Opin Infect Dis 2019;32:372–9.

470. Radonovich LJ Jr, Yanke R, Cheng J, Bender B. Diminished speech intelligibility associated with certain types of respirators worn by healthcare workers. J Occup Environ Hyg 2010;7:63–70.

471. Law BHY, Cheung PY, Aziz K, Schmölzer GM. Effect of COVID-19 Precautions on neonatal resuscitation practice: a balance between healthcare provider safety, infection control, and effective neonatal care. Front Pediatr 2020;8:478.

472. Seale H, Leem J-S, Gallard J, et al. "The cookie monster muffler": Perceptions and behaviours of hospital healthcare workers around the use of masks and respirators in the hospital setting. Int J Infect Control 2015;11:i1. doi: 10.3396/IJIC.v11i1.006.15.

473. Baskett PJ, Steen PA, Bossaert L; European Resuscitation Council. European Resuscitation Council guidelines for resuscitation 2005. Section 8. The ethics of resuscitation and end-of-life decisions. Resuscitation 2005;67 (Suppl 1):S171–80.

474. Harvey ME, Pattison HM. The impact of a father's presence during newborn resuscitation: a qualitative interview study with healthcare professionals. BMJ Open 2013;3:e002547.

475. Jabre P, Belpomme V, Azoulay E, et al. Family presence during cardiopulmonary resuscitation. N Engl J Med 2013;368:1008–18.

476. Jabre P, Tazarourte K, Azoulay E, et al. Offering the opportunity for family to be present during cardiopulmonary resuscitation: 1-year assessment. Intensive Care Med 2014;40:981–7.

477. Trevisanuto D, Moschino L, Doglioni N, Roehr CC, Gervasi MT, Baraldi E. Neonatal resuscitation where the mother has a suspected or confirmed novel coronavirus (SARS-CoV-2) infection: Suggestion for a pragmatic action plan. Neonatology 2020;117:133–40.

478. Yoxall CW, Ayers S, Sawyer A, et al. Providing immediate neonatal care and resuscitation at birth beside the mother: clinicians' views, a qualitative study. BMJ Open 2015;5:e008494.

479. Katheria AC, Sorkhi SR, Hassen K, Faksh A, Ghorishi Z, Poeltler D. Acceptability of bedside resuscitation with intact umbilical cord to clinicians and patients' families in the United States. Front Pediatr 2018;6:100.

480. Wyllie JP, Wyckoff MH, de Almeida MF, et al. Family presence during neonatal resuscitation. International Liaison Committee on Resuscitation (ILCOR) Neonatal Life Support Task Force, Nov 2020. Available from: http://ilcor.org

481. Dainty KN, Atkins DL, Breckwoldt J, et al; International Liaison Committee on Resuscitation's (ILCOR) Pediatric; Neonatal Life Support Task Force; Education, Implementation and Teams Task Force. Family presence during resuscitation in paediatric and neonatal cardiac arrest: A systematic review. Resuscitation 2021;162:20-34.

482. Brei BK, Sawyer T, Umoren R, et al; National Emergency Airway Registry for Neonates (NEAR4NEOS) investigators. Associations between family presence and neonatal intubation outcomes: a report from the National Emergency Airway Registry for Neonates: NEAR4NEOS. Arch Dis Child Fetal Neonatal Ed 2021:fetalneonatal-2020-319709. [Epub ahead of print].

483. Zehnder E, Law BHY, Schmölzer GM. Does parental presence affect workload during neonatal resuscitation? Arch Dis Child Fetal Neonatal Ed 2020;105:559–61.

484. Arnold L, Sawyer A, Rabe H, et al. Parents' first moments with their very preterm babies: a qualitative study. BMJ Open 2013;3:e002487.

485. Abel F, Bajaj Y, Wyatt M, Wallis C. The successful use of the nasopharyngeal airway in Pierre Robin sequence: an 11-year experience. Arch Dis Child 2012;97:331–4.

486. Parhizkar N, Saltzman B, Grote K, et al. Nasopharyngeal airway for management of airway obstruction in infants with micrognathia. Cleft Palate Craniofac J 2011;48:478–82.

487. Roberts K, Whalley H, Bleetman A. The Nasopharyngeal airway: Dispelling myths and establishing the facts. Emerg Med J 2005;22:394–6.

488. Shen CM, Soong WJ, Jeng MJ, et al. Nasopharyngeal tract length measurement in infants. Acta Paediatr Taiwan 2002;43:82–5.

489. Heaf DP, Helms PJ, Dinwiddie R, et al. Nasopharyngeal airways in Pierre Robin Syndrome. J Pediatr 1982;100:698–703.

490. Roberts K, Porter K. How do you size a nasopharyngeal airway? Resuscitation 2003;56:19–23.

491. O'Shea JE, Loganathan P, Thio M, Kamlin COF, Davis PG. Analysis of unsuccessful intubations in neonates using videolaryngoscopy recordings. Arch Dis Child Fetal Neonatal Ed 2018;103:F408–12.

492. O'Shea JE, Thio M, Kamlin CO, et al. Videolaryngoscopy to teach neonatal intubation: A randomized trial. Pediatrics 2015;136:912–9.

493. Parmekar S, Arnold JL, Anselmo C, et al. Mind the gap: can videolaryngoscopy bridge the competency gap in neonatal endotracheal intubation among pediatric trainees? A randomized controlled study. J Perinatol 2017;37:979–83.

494. Kirolos S, O'Shea JE. Comparison of conventional and videolaryngoscopy blades in neonates. Arch Dis Child Fetal Neonatal Ed 2020;105:94–7.

495. Upton CJ, Milner AD. Endotracheal resuscitation of neonates using a rebreathing bag. Arch Dis Child 1991;66:39–42.

496. Hey E, Hull D. Lung function at birth in babies developing respiratory distress. J Obstet Gynaecol Br Commonw 1971;78:1137–46.

497. O'Donnell CP, Kamlin CO, Davis PG, Morley CJ. Endotracheal intubation attempts during neonatal resuscitation: success rates, duration and adverse effects. Pediatrics 2006;117:e16–21.

498. Fayoux P, Devisme L, Merrot O, Marciniak B. Determination of endotracheal tube size in a perinatal population: an anatomical and experimental study. Anesthesiology 2006;104:954–60.

499. Gill I, O'Donnell CP. Vocal cord guides on neonatal endotracheal tubes. Arch Dis Child Fetal Neonatal Ed 2014;99:F344.

500. Leung C. Optimal insertion depth for endotracheal tubes in extremely low-birth-weight infants. Pediatr Crit Care Med 2018;19:328–31.

501. Kempley ST, Moreiras JW, Petrone FL. Endotracheal tube length for neonatal intubation. Resuscitation 2008;77:369–73.

502. Loew A, Thibeault DW. A new and safe method to control the depth of endotracheal intubation in neonates. Pediatrics 1974;54:506–8.

503. Kamlin COF, O'Donnell CPF, Davis PG, et al. Colorimetric end-tidal carbon dioxide detectors in the delivery room: strengths and limitations. A case report. J Pediatr 2005;147:547–8.

504. Doss A. Resuscitation of the newborn. Br Med J 1964;2:1331–41.

505. Hosono S, Inami I, Fujita H, et al. A role of end-tidal CO2 monitoring for assessment of tracheal intubations in very low birth weight infants during neonatal resuscitation at birth. J Perinat Med 2009;37:79–84.

506. Roberts WA, Maniscalco WM, Cohen AR, et al. The use of capnography for recognition of esophageal intubation in the neonatal intensive care unit. Pediatr Pulmonol 1995;19:262–8.

507. Aziz HF, Martin JB, Moore JJ. The pediatric disposable end-tidal carbon dioxide detector role in endotracheal intubation in newborns. J Perinatol 1999;19:110–3.

508. Hughes SM, Blake BL, Woods SL, Lehmann CU. False-positive results on colorimetric carbon dioxide analysis in neonatal resuscitation: potential for serious patient harm. J Perinatol 2007;27:800–1.

509. Meyer WW, Lind J. The ductus venosus and the mechanism of its closure. Arch Dis Child 1966;41:597–605.

510. Heinild S, Søndergaard T, Tudvad F. Bone marrow infusions in childhood: experiences from a thousand infusions. J Pediatr 1947;30:400–11.

511. Bohn D. Intraosseous vascular access: from the archives to the ABC. Crit Care Med 1999;27:1053–4.

512. Abe KK, Blum GT, Yamamoto LG. Intraosseous is faster and easier than umbilical venous catheterization in newborn emergency vascular access models. Am J Emerg Med 2000;18:126–9.

513. Vidal R, Kissoon N, Gayle M. Compartment syndrome following intraosseous infusion. Pediatrics 1993;91:1201–2.

514. Oesterlie GE, Petersen KK, Knudsen L, et al. Crural amputation of a newborn as a consequence of intraosseous needle insertion and calcium infusion. Pediatr Emerg Care 2014;30:413–4.

515. La Flece FR, Slepin MJ, Vargasa J, et al. Iatrogenic bilateral tibial fractures after intraosseous infusion attempts in a 3-month-old infant. Ann Emerg Med 1989;18:1099–101.

516. Chawla S, Amaram A, Gopal SP, Natarajan G. Safety and efficacy of Trans-warmer mattress for preterm neonates: results of a randomized controlled trial. J Perinatol 2011;31:780–4.

517. Almeida PG, Chandley J, Davis J, Harrigan RC. Use of the heated gel mattress and its impact on admission temperature of very low birthweight infants. Adv Neonatal Care 2009;9:34–9.

518. Thomas MR, Yoxall CW, Weeks AD, Duley L. Providing newborn resuscitation at the mother's bedside: assessing the safety, usability and acceptability of a mobile trolley. BMC Pediatr 2014;14:135.

519. Hawkes CP, Oni OA, Dempsey EM, et al. Potential hazard of the Neopuff T piece resuscitator in the absence of flow limitation. Arch Dis Child Fetal Neonatal Ed 2009;94:F461–3.

520. Schilleman K, Schmölzer GM, Kamlin OC, et al. Changing gas flow during neonatal resuscitation: a manikin study. Resuscitation 2011;82:920–4.

521. Finer NN, Rich WD. Unintentional variation in positive end expiratory pressure during resuscitation with a T-piece resuscitator. Resuscitation 2011;82:717–9.

522. Dawson JA, Schmölzer GM, Kamlin CO, et al. Oxygenation with T-piece versus self-inflating bag for ventilation of extremely preterm infants at birth: a randomized controlled trial. J Pediatr 2011;158:912–8.e1-2.

523. Szyld E, Aguilar A, Musante GA, et al; Delivery Room Ventilation Devices Trial Group. Comparison of devices for newborn ventilation in the delivery room. J Pediatr 2014;165:234–9.e3.

524. Hawkes CP, Ryan CA, Dempsey EM. Comparison of the T piece resuscitator with other neonatal manual ventilation devices: a qualitative review. Resuscitation 2012;83:797–802.

525. O'Donnell CP, Davis PG, Lau R, Dargaville PA, Doyle LW, Morley CJ. Neonatal resuscitation 2: an evaluation of manual ventilation devices and face masks. Arch Dis Child Fetal Neonatal Ed 2005;90:F392–6.

526. Kattwinkel J, Stewart C, Walsh B, Gurka M, Paget-Brown A. Responding to compliance changes in a lung model during manual ventilation: perhaps volume, rather than pressure, should be displayed. Pediatrics 2009;123:e465–70.

527. Klingenberg C, Wheeler KI, Davis PG, et al. A practical guide to neonatal volume guarantee ventilation. J Perinatol 2011;31:575–85.

528. Schmölzer GM, Poulton DA, Dawson JA, Kamlin CO, Morley CJ, Davis PG. Assessment of flow waves and colorimetric CO2 detector for endotracheal tube placement during neonatal resuscitation. Resuscitation 2011;82:307–12.

529. Field D, Milner AD, Hopkin IE. Efficiency of manual resuscitators at birth. Arch Dis Child 1986;61:300–2.

530. Oddie S, Wyllie J, Scally A. Use of self-inflating bags for neonatal resuscitation. Resuscitation 2005;67:109–12.

531. Ainsworth SB, Humphreys R, Stewart L. The pressure is on! The danger of a broken blow off valve on a bag valve mask. Arch Dis Child Fetal Neonatal Ed 2006;91:F233.

532. Cushing P. Mis-assembly of adult and paediatric manual resuscitators. Resuscitation 2002;55:347–8.

533. te Pas AB, Lopriore E, Dito I, Morley CJ, Walther FJ. Humidified and heated air during stabilization at birth improves temperature in preterm infants. Pediatrics 2010;125:e1427–32.

534. Meyer MP, Hou D, Ishrar NN, Dito I, te Pas AB. Initial respiratory support with cold, dry gas versus heated humidified gas and admission temperature of preterm infants. J Pediatr 2015;166:245–50.e1.

535. McGrory L, Owen LS, Thio M, et al. A randomized trial of conditioned or unconditioned gases for stabilizing preterm infants at birth. J Pediatr 2018;193:47–53.

536. Murphy MC, De Angelis L, McCarthy LK, O'Donnell CPF. Comparison of infant heart rate assessment by auscultation, ECG and oximetry in the delivery room. Arch Dis Child Fetal Neonatal Ed 2018;103:F490–2.

537. Kamlin CO, Dawson JA, O'Donnell CP, et al. Accuracy of pulse oximetry measurement of heart rate of newborn infants in the delivery room. J Pediatr 2008;152:756–60.

538. Kamlin CO, O'Donnell CP, Everest NJ, Davis PG, Morley CJ. Accuracy of clinical assessment of infant heart rate in the delivery room. Resuscitation 2006;71:319–21.

539. O'Donnell CPF, Kamlin COF, Davis PG, Morley CJ. Obtaining pulse oximetry data in neonates: a randomised crossover study of sensor application techniques. Arch Dis Child Fetal Neonatal Ed 2005;90:F84–5.

540. Narayen IC, Smit M, van Zwet EW, Dawson JA, Blom NA, te Pas AB. Low signal quality pulse oximetry measurements in newborn infants are reliable for oxygen saturation but underestimate heart rate. Acta Paediatr 2015;104:e158–63.

541. Anton O, Fernandez R, Rendon-Morales E, Aviles-Espinosa R, Jordan H, Rabe H. Heart rate monitoring in newborn babies: a systematic review. Neonatology 2019;116:199–210.

542. Johnson PA, Cheung PY, Lee TF, O'Reilly M, Schmölzer GM. Novel technologies for heart rate assessment during neonatal resuscitation at birth - A systematic review. Resuscitation 2019;143:196–207.

543. Mizumoto H, Tomotaki S, Shibata H, et al. Electrocardiogram shows reliable heart rates much earlier than pulse oximetry during neonatal resuscitation. Pediatr Int 2012;54:205–7.

544. Iglesias B, Rodrí Guez MAJ, Aleo E, Criado E, Martí Nez-Orgado J, Arruza L. 3-lead electrocardiogram is more reliable than pulse oximetry to detect bradycardia during stabilisation at birth of very preterm infants. Arch Dis Child Fetal Neonatal Ed 2018;103:F233–7.

545. Sillers L, Handley SC, James JR, Foglia EE. Pulseless electrical activity complicating neonatal resuscitation. Neonatology 2019;115:95–98.

546. Zareen Z, Hawkes CP, Krickan ER, Dempsey EM, Ryan CA. In vitro comparison of neonatal suction catheters using simulated 'pea soup' meconium. Arch Dis Child Fetal Neonatal Ed 2013;98:F241–3.

547. Kelleher J, Bhat R, Salas AA, et al. Oronasopharyngeal suction versus wiping of the mouth and nose at birth: a randomised equivalency trial. Lancet 2013;382:326–30.

548. Bancalari A, Díaz V, Araneda H. Effects of pharyngeal suction on the arterial oxygen saturation and heart rate in healthy newborns delivered by elective cesarean section. J Neonatal Perinatal Med 2019;12:271–6.

Useful links

The Advanced Resusciation of the Newborn Infant (ARNI) course has been developed for NLS providers who have ongoing involvement in neonatal care and are working in a capacity where they may be called on to be a key member of a resuscitation team or provide intensive care, however briefly, to any baby from their birth until discharge home.

Become an RCUK NLS Instructor

Exceptional candidates may be nominated by the faculty to become an NLS instructor. The Course Director and faculty must support the nomination and provide a detailed statement of support to RCUK.

To be successfully put forward as an Instructor Potential (IP), the candidate must be a (statutory/ voluntary) registered healthcare professional with regular ongoing hands-on care of the newborn and active participation in resuscitation at birth.

Candidates must demonstrate excellent core knowledge of the course content, excellent and safe practical application of skills, and have exceptional communication skills.

Potential instructors should be confident, flexible, adaptable, interactive, supportive and enthusiastic. If successfully nominated, the candidate would need to undertake an RCUK Generic Instructor Course (GIC) and complete two supported supervised teaching practices as an Instructor Candidate (IC).

More information regarding the GIC can be accessed here: https://www.resus.org.uk/training-courses/instructorcourses/gic-generic-instructor-course.

Benefits of becoming an instructor for RCUK:

You will join the RCUK community of practice with opportunities for portfolio development and ongoing access to the latest research and resuscitation practices.

You will become a subject matter expert, and your instructor qualification will be recognised throughout the UK and Europe.

As an instructor, you'll be eligible to attend RCUK's popular Instructor Days, and you will

also, receive free RCUK Associate membership.

Being an active NLS instructor means you are also an NLS provider.

For more information on how you can become an RCUK NLS instructor, please speak to the Course Director before or on the day of your course.

Resuscitation Council UK Guidelines
Read all of the 2021 guidelines:
resus.org.uk/rcukgl21

Lifesaver and Lifesaver VR apps
Teach your friends and family lifesaving skills anytime, anywhere:
resus.org.uk/rcuklifesaver

iResus app
Get RCUK guidelines on the go:
resus.org.uk/rcukiresus

e-Lifesaver
Bring lifesaving training to your non-clinical staff:
resus.org.uk/rcukworkplace

Resuscitation Council UK courses
See all of the courses available:
resus.org.uk/rcukcourses

Follow us on Twitter
@ResusCouncilUK
twitter.com/ResusCouncilUK

RCUK membership
Get involved and join our community:
resus.org.uk/rcukmembers

Like us on Facebook
facebook.com/ResuscitationCouncilUK

Notes

Notes

Notes

Notes